INTERPROFESSIONAL LEADERSHIP FOR NURSES

INTERPROFESSIONAL LEADERSHIP FOR NURSES

Mastering Knowledge, Skills, and Attitudes for Success

CAROL SAVRIN and **JESSE HONSKY**, Editors

Case Western Reserve University

cognella®

SAN DIEGO

Bassim Hamadeh, CEO and Publisher

Amanda Martin, Publisher

Amy Smith, Senior Project Editor

Jeanine Rees, Production Editor

Jess Estrella, Senior Graphic Designer

Kylie Bartolome, Licensing Specialist

Natalie Piccotti, Director of Marketing

Kassie Graves, Senior Vice President, Editorial

cognella® | ACADEMIC PUBLISHING

3970 Sorrento Valley Blvd., Ste. 500, San Diego, CA 92121

BRIEF CONTENTS

Jesse Honsky, DNP, MPH, RN, PHNA-BC

*Georgia L. Narsavage, PhD, APRN, CNS-BC, FAAN, FNAP, ATSF, and
Catherine S. Koppelman, MSN, RN, R, NEA, CNO, Executive Coach*

*Rita Sfiligoj, DNP, MPA, RN, Shannon Wong, MSN, RN, CPNP, Jesse Honsky,
DNP, MPH, RN, PHNA-BC, and Carol Savrin, DNP, RN, CPNP, R, FNP-BC,
FAANP, FNAP*

*Kristina Banks, DNP, APRN, CPNP-PC, and Mary de Haan, MSN, RN,
ACNS-BC, CNE*

*Marie D. Grosh, DNP, APRN-CNP, LNHA, Carli A. Carnish, DNP, RN,
APRN-CNP, and Carol Savrin, DNP, CPNP, R, CNP-BC, FAANP, FNAP*

Janna Draine Kinney, DNP, RN, CCRN, and Me'Chelle Hayes, MSN, RN, FNP-BC

Carol Savrin, DNP, RN, CPNP, R, FNP-BC, FAANP, FNAP, and Jesse Honsky, DNP, MPH, RN, PHNA-BC

Deborah Lindell, DNP, MSN, RN, CNE, ANEF, FAAN, and Beverly Capper, DNP, MSN, RNC-NIC

Carol Savrin, DNP, CPNP, R, FNP-BC, FAANP, FANP, and Catherine Demko, PhD

DETAILED CONTENTS

Chapter 2   Leadership Style

Georgia L. Narsavage, PhD, APRN, CNS-BC, FAAN, FNAP, ATSF, and Catherine S. Koppelman, MSN, RN, R, NEA, CNO, Executive Coach

Chapter 3   Communication

Rita Sfiligoj, DNP, MPA, RN, Shannon Wong, MSN, RN, CPNP, Jesse Honsky, DNP, MPH, RN, PHNA-BC, and Carol Savrin, DNP, RN, CPNP, R, FNP-BC, FAANP, FNAP

Chapter 4   Effective Role Performance

Kristina Banks, DNP, APRN, CPNP-PC, and Mary de Haan, MSN, RN, ACNS-BC, CNE

Chapter 5   Roles and Responsibilities

Marie D. Grosh, DNP, APRN-CNP, LNHA, Carli A. Carnish, DNP, RN, APRN-CNP, and Carol Savrin, DNP, CPNP, R, CNP-BC, FAANP, FNAP

Chapter 6 Respect

Janna Draine Kinney, DNP, RN, CCRN, and Me'Chelle Hayes, MSN, RN, FNP-BC

Chapter 7 Conflict Management

Carol Savrin, DNP, RN, CPNP, R, FNP-BC, FAANP, FNAP, and Jesse Honsky, DNP, MPH, RN, PHNA-BC

Chapter 8   Personal Health, Resilience, and Well-Being

Deborah Lindell, DNP, MSN, RN, CNE, ANEF, FAAN, and Beverly Capper,
DNP, MSN, RNC-NIC

Chapter 9   Direct Observation of Team Interactions

*Carol Savrin, DNP, CPNP, R, FNP-BC, FAANP, FANP,
and Catherine Demko, PhD*

REVIEWERS

Ericka K. Waidley, PhD, MS, MSN, BSN
Linfield University-School of Nursing, Portland, Oregon

Daniel Pesut, PhD, RN, FAAN
University of Minnesota School of Nursing

Carrie Hintz, DNP, PhD(c), RN, CEN, CNML
University of Nevada, Reno—Orvis School of Nursing

Arielle St. Romain, DNP, RN, CNEcl
University of Louisiana at Lafayette

Anne Walsh, MMSc, PA-C, DFAAPA
Clinical Associate Professor, PA Studies, Chapman University,
Crean College of Health and Behavioral Sciences

Sharonda Johnson, MSN, RN
University of Louisiana at Lafayette

CONTRIBUTORS

Kristina Banks, DNP, APRN, CPNP-PC
Instructor, Frances Payne Bolton School of Nursing,
Case Western Reserve University

Beverly Capper, DNP, MSN, RNC-NIC
Assistant Professor, Frances Payne Bolton School of Nursing,
Case Western Reserve University

Carli A. Carnish, DNP, RN, APRN-CNP
Assistant Professor, Frances Payne Bolton School of Nursing,
Case Western Reserve University

Catherine Demko, PhD
Associate Professor, School of Dental Medicine,
Case Western Reserve University

Mary de Haan, MSN, RN, ACNS-BC, CNE
Instructor, Frances Payne Bolton School of Nursing,
Case Western Reserve University

Marie Grosh DNP, ARPN-CNP, LNHA
Assistant Professor, Frances Payne Bolton School of Nursing,
Case Western Reserve University

Me'Chelle Hayes, MSN, RN, FNP-BC
Instructor, Frances Payne Bolton School of Nursing,
Case Western Reserve University

Jesse Honsky, DNP, MPH, RN, PHNA-BC
Assistant Professor, Frances Payne Bolton School of Nursing,
Case Western Reserve University

Janna Draine Kinney, DNP, RN, CCRN
Instructor, Frances Payne Bolton School of Nursing,
Case Western Reserve University

Deborah Lindell, DNP, MSN, RN, CNE, ANEF, FAAN
Professor, Frances Payne Bolton School of Nursing,
Case Western Reserve University

Catherine S. Koppelman, MSN, RN,R, NEA, CNO, Executive Coach
Former Chief Nursing Officer, University Hospitals, Cleveland, OH

Georgia L. Narsavage, PhD, APRN, CNS-BC, FAAN, FNAP, ATSF
Professor Emerita and Former Dean, School of Nursing,
West Virginia University, Morgantown, West Virginia;
Former Director of Interprofessional Education for
Health Sciences, West Virginia University

Carol Savrin, DNP, RN, CPNP,R, FNP-BC, FAANP, FNAP
Associate Professor, Frances Payne Bolton School of Nursing

Rita Sfiligoj, DNP, MPA, RN
Assistant Professor, Frances Payne Bolton School of Nursing,
Case Western Reserve University

Shannon Wong, MSN, RN, CPNP
Instructor, Frances Payne Bolton School of Nursing,
Case Western Reserve University

Special thanks goes to Ellen Luebbers, MD, who contributed to the development of the DOTI.

CHAPTER 1

Interprofessional Collaboration and Leadership

Jesse Honsky, DNP, MPH, RN, PHNA-BC

INTRODUCTION: WHAT ARE INTERPROFESSIONAL COLLABORATION AND LEADERSHIP?

This handbook will equip you with some skills and tools you may need as you transition into your new nursing role and help you feel more confident taking on a leadership role in the interprofessional team. Leadership and teamwork may seem like easy concepts to understand and often appear just as plain common sense. However, understanding a concept does not necessarily mean you will feel prepared to apply it when a situation arises. For example, many of us know how we are supposed to deliver difficult news to a patient: We should sit down for the conversation, address the patient directly, express empathy, and use clear language. Now think back to one of the first times a patient asked you a difficult question that you did not know how to answer. How did you respond? Did you immediately know how to answer the question? Were you able to deliver the answer without hesitation? Did you feel nervous or uncomfortable? What words did you use? How did you respond with your body language? Have you become more comfortable addressing similar questions since that time? The intentional practice of and reflection on communication skills can hone the skills needed to communicate effectively with patients and other members of the health care team. Additional skills associated with leadership and teamwork can be developed intentionally as well. In this book, we identify some of the skills, knowledge, and attitudes most important for new nurses and nurses transitioning into advanced roles.

INTERPROFESSIONAL COLLABORATIVE PRACTICE

Interprofessional collaborative practice is when health care professionals (HCPs) from different professions work with patients, families, caregivers, communities, and each other to provide high-quality care (Interprofessional Education Collaborative, 2016; World Health Organization, 2010). The patient, family, and community are essential members of the interprofessional team, along with professionals such as nurses, advanced practice nurses (APRNs), counselors, dentists, pharmacists, physicians, physician assistants/associates[1] (PAs), physical therapists, speech-language pathologists, occupational therapists, social workers, nursing aids, surgical technologists, and administrative staff, just to name a few.

When working on an interprofessional team, we need to not only take into account our competence as a nurse but also the competence level of the team. In health care, we focus primarily on the competence of the individual. Individuals earn their grades and degrees and then are licensed and certified. We typically assess job performance individually, yet we know that ineffective

---

[1] In 2021 the American Academy of Physician Associates (AAPA) voted to begin using "physician associate" instead of physician assistant as the official title for PAs. The official title has not been adopted in every U.S. state, so both titles are still in use. For more information see the AAPA website: https://www.aapa.com.org/title-change/.

teams are often the source of inadequate care and medical errors (Lingard, 2016). It is simply not enough to be individually competent. Nurses and other HCPs must understand and practice how to work on a competent team and take collective responsibility for the team's functioning. See Table 1.1 for some of the myths and truths about competent health care teams observed through extensive research on how teams work together.

TABLE 1.1   **Myths and Truths About Health Care Teams**

Myths	Truths
"If we each did our job properly, then this team would be effective."	"Competent individuals can form an incompetent team."
"If we understood each other's roles, then this team would be competent."	"Teams can be competent even when one team member is incompetent."
"If we had clear leadership and accountability, then this team would function well."	'An incompetent team member can derail one team, but another carries on around [them]."
"If we all just focused on the patient, then this team would work smoothly."	"The same team can be competent in one situation and incompetent in another."

Source: Lingard (2016, pp. S19, S20).

The myths in Table 1.1 are described not because they are entirely wrong but because they are incomplete and reflect an oversimplification of how teams work. Understanding the roles of each team member is an important step to helping a team function well; however, sometimes roles are not distinct, and they can overlap and shift (Lingard, 2016). All members of the team can play a role in patient education. If everyone on the team assumes that someone else is doing the education because it is their role, the patient may not get the information they need. Conversely, if every team member educates the patient but does not coordinate with the other team members, the information could be incomplete or overwhelming. HCPs need to understand each other's roles and how their roles overlap and that there can be ambiguity when it comes to some tasks and functions.

The truths in Table 1.1 speak to how teams are more than just the sum of their parts. Simply doing your job to the best of your ability in isolation will not result in effective teamwork; communication, trust, and shared experience among team members are also needed. A team is more than just a group of people who work together. A team consists of "two or more people who interact dynamically, interdependently, and adaptively toward a common and valued goal; have specific roles or functions; and have a time-limited membership" (Agency for Healthcare Research and Quality, n.d. para. 8). To be a team individuals must communicate and collaborate, and their ability to do their work relies on the work of other team members. In health care, teams may be consistent, like a team that works in a primary care clinic together daily, or may frequently change, like on a hospital floor, when the team changes with each shift. Conversely, a group may have a shared goal, but individuals work independently of each other, assuming that the work is coordinated by others (Armstead et al., 2016). This assumption and isolation from other members of the group can lead to gaps and fragmentation in care.

Interprofessional collaborative practice has the potential to address all aspects of the Quintuple Aim to improve patient health outcomes, the patient experience, health equity, HCP job satisfaction, and lower health care costs. The Quintuple Aim grew out of the Institute for Healthcare Improvements (IHI) Triple Aim, as a framework to help health care systems improve their performance, it started focusing on improving population health (patient outcomes), patient experience, and lowering costs

(Berwick et al., 2008; Institute for Healthcare Improvement, n.d.). In 2014, Bodenheimer and Sinsky (2014) proposed the Quadruple Aim, adding HCP well-being to the framework, and in 2021 the framework was expanded to include health equity (Nundy et al., 2022; Itchhaporia, 2021 pp. 2263 see Figure 1.1).

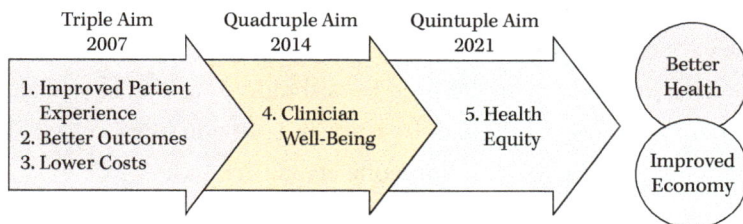

Triple Aim 2007	Quadruple Aim 2014	Quintuple Aim 2021	
1. Improved Patient Experience 2. Better Outcomes 3. Lower Costs	4. Clinician Well-Being	5. Health Equity	Better Health Improved Economy

FIGURE 1.1   Evolution of the Quintuple Aim.

By working better together, HCPs have the potential to improve the lives of their patients and the greater community and can improve their own job satisfaction and relationships with coworkers.

Leadership

In simplest terms, leadership is how an individual influences a group of people to achieve a shared goal (Northouse, 2022). Nurses can lead in many different ways. A nurse may be considered a leader because of their formal role as a nurse manager or executive within a health care organization. They may also have an informal leadership role because of their expertise and because they are trusted by their coworkers.

The purpose of this book is to provide you with the knowledge, skills, and attitudes you will need to take on both formal and informal leadership roles in your future health care team while taking care of patients. An important aspect of interprofessional collaborative practice is shared leadership, the idea that all team members have the ability and are allowed to influence the team (Dow et al., 2015). While there may be a formal leader of the health care team, typically this is the provider, such as a physician, APRN, or PA—all team members who can lead based on the circumstances and their specific skill set. For example, suppose a patient is adhering to their treatment plan but is still struggling with activities of daily living; the occupational therapist may need to step up to lead the team in order to find the best solution for the patient. The team should recognize and respect the expertise that the occupational therapist brings to the table. All interprofessional team members should develop the skills to step up when needed to lead the team and provide support to their team members when it is someone else's turn to lead.

Hierarchy and Power in Health Care

True interprofessional collaboration and shared leadership can be challenging to achieve in health care because of its traditionally hierarchical structure and the power differentials between individuals of different professions. Interprofessional collaboration seeks to flatten the hierarchy and to engage all team members, including the patient, in shared decision-making (Bachynsky, 2020; Nelson et al., 2014).

Hierarchy and imbalance of power in health care can have negative impacts on the health care team; for example, individuals working in rigid hierarchies may be less likely to speak up if they have differing opinions or have concerns about a medical error. Hierarchies can result in bullying and feelings of powerlessness (Essex et al., 2023). Individuals may feel they have less power for many reasons, such as their professional role, their rank or length of service, or social status.

HCPs do not always perceive interprofessional collaboration in the same way. In general, nurses tend to perceive interprofessional collaboration more positively and desire to see more collaboration, specifically by expanding nursing autonomy. In contrast, physicians tend to believe that good collaboration already exists (Sollami et al., 2015). HCPs, who are not nurses or physicians, also report a relationship between autonomy and collaboration. Those with lower levels of autonomy felt their professional expertise and knowledge were not respected, which can impede collaboration (Seaton et al., 2021). The team leader may think collaboration is working well when they can direct the team and each member follows orders. However, the other team members may be resentful that they are not consulted on the treatment plan, are not allowed to use their professional judgment, and do not feel comfortable talking about their concerns with the group. Thinking that your team is good at collaboration is not enough; your team should share their expectations and perceptions with each other. A strong leader can create an environment in which people feel comfortable discussing the functioning of their team.

OVERVIEW OF THE HANDBOOK

The authors selected the topics for each chapter of this handbook to align with the skills that are needed to lead an interprofessional team effectively and with competencies identified by the American Association of Colleges of Nursing (AACN, 2021) that are essential to nursing practice at both the entry-level and advanced levels. In this handbook, entry-level nursing education refers to bachelor of science in nursing (BSN) and prelicensure programs. Advanced-level education refers to graduate-level education in nursing such as a master of science in nursing (MSN) or doctor of nursing practice (DNP) degree. You may choose to focus on the content that best applies to your education level and future level of practice. To simplify the language, we refer to practicing nurses with a BSN or other entry-level degree as registered nurses (RN). The term *advanced-level nurses* applies to nurses who have earned a graduate degree and work as an APRN or in other advanced nursing roles that require further education, such as nurse executives, advanced public health nurses, or nurse educators.

Each chapter begins by listing the AACN competencies and sub-competencies that are relevant to the topic to identify how this content addresses the skills essential to nursing practice. The authors of each chapter then describe important concepts and terms and share how they are relevant to nursing practice, interprofessional collaboration, and leadership through real-world examples. Finally, each chapter provides activities to help you better understand and apply the concepts described. The research and literature around leadership are extensive, but this book is not intended to be all-encompassing. Instead, it focuses on the skills, knowledge, and attitudes that may be most helpful for new nurses (both entry and advanced levels), when working with an interprofessional team.

Chapter 2: Leadership Style

This chapter introduces some key leadership concepts as they apply to nurses in direct patient care roles. In this chapter, you will find information and strategies to help you build your leadership style to set the foundation for professional and personal growth throughout your nursing career.

Chapter 3: Communication

Good communication is essential to the interprofessional team. This chapter provides concrete tools that HCPs can use with each other and with patients in order to maintain clear lines of communication. It includes communication among individuals and through the use of technology. In addition to sharing common communication tools, it explores some of the barriers to communication and strategies to address those barriers.

Chapter 4: Effective Role Performance

To be influential leaders on an interprofessional team, nurses must perform their roles effectively and understand how to help the team work effectively together. This chapter discusses how a just culture, team roles, team dynamics, and expertise can enhance individual and team performance.

Chapter 5: Roles and Responsibilities

The chapter about roles and responsibilities differs from the effective role performance chapter in that it focuses on understanding the roles and responsibilities of each health care team member. This includes understanding where they differ and where they may overlap. In addition, this chapter provides information on how nurses can better articulate their role on the interprofessional team to others.

Chapter 6: Respect

Respect is essential to building a high-functioning team. For a team to work well together, each individual must feel valued and comfortable speaking up to the group. This chapter outlines issues around respect, integrity, incivility, bullying, implicit bias, and microaggressions and how nurses and HCPs can foster respect and create a positive working environment for all team members, including patients.

Chapter 7: Conflict Management

Conflict is inevitable in health care and when working on an interprofessional team. A good leader does not avoid or minimize conflict but learns how to manage conflict. When managed appropriately, conflict can be a positive experience for a team and may result in better patient and team outcomes. This chapter introduces concepts and strategies that are useful when navigating conflict on interprofessional teams, including psychological safety, conflict management styles, and tips for working through conflict at individual and organizational levels.

Chapter 8: Personal Health, Resilience, and Well-Being

A career in the health care field can be very demanding and high pressure. As a leader, learning to take care of yourself and modeling self-care to your team is important. Establishing self-care routines early in your career can help you to navigate the complex health care environment better. In addition, understanding the systems-level issues that impact HCP well-being is essential for nurses to lead change to improve the health care work environment. This chapter provides concrete strategies for promoting self-care and reducing burnout among nurses and other HCPs. The chapter addresses both individual and systems-level activities.

Chapter 9: Direct Observation of Team Interactions

The Direct Observations of Team Interactions (DOTI) is an instrument used to assess how well a team is functioning based on their interactions. This instrument is a useful resource to assess how well your team is performing and as a framework to understand better *how* effective teams function. This chapter provides more detail about DOTI and how to use it in clinical and simulation settings.

TAKING AN ACTIVE ROLE IN YOUR LEARNING

This handbook is another tool to help you on your career journey. While reading, consider your personal learning needs and professional goals. Learners should take an active role in their education and be invested in their learning to meet the competencies identified by the AACN (2023). In addition, this prepares you to continue as a lifelong learner. Health care is an ever-changing field that requires ongoing education and skill development. You can assess your progress toward the competencies through the activities in this book, personal reflection, and discussions with faculty, preceptors, and peers. We hope you find information and strategies in this book that serve you well as you transition into your professional nursing role.

KEY POINTS

- The skills of teamwork and leadership require intentional practice and development.
- HCPs must be individually competent and take responsibility for the team's competence.
- An effective interprofessional team will share leadership among team members. Team members should be prepared to step up to leaders when appropriate and be supportive of the leadership of other team members.
- Hierarchy and power imbalance in health care can contribute to a negative working environment and harm patient care. Interprofessional collaboration seeks to flatten those hierarchies and engage all team members.
- The topics covered in this book align with AACN competencies and the skills needed to lead interprofessional teams. As you read through the text, identify the knowledge, skills, and attitudes most useful to your learning and professional development.

COMMON ABBREVIATIONS AND TERMS

In this book, many abbreviations and terms are used frequently across chapters. To avoid defining the same abbreviation or term multiple times, we introduce each one once, then use it consistently throughout the book. We have listed the most common abbreviations and terms in this book for easy reference:

- **Advanced-level nurse**: an APRN, or a nurse who has completed either a master's or doctoral degree in nursing

- **APRN**: Advanced practice registered nurse (i.e., clinical nurse specialist, nurse anesthetist, nurse-midwife, nurse practitioner)
- **EHR**: Electronic health record
- **HCP**: Health care professional
- **NP**: Nurse practitioner
- **Nurse**: Inclusive of entry-level prepared nurses, RN, and advanced-level nurses
- **PA**: Physician assistant or physician associate
- **Provider**: Referring to advanced practice providers (i.e., APRNs, physicians, and PAs)
- **RN**: Registered nurse who has completed a nursing program that prepared for them entry-level nursing practice (e.g., BSN)

ACTIVITIES

Activity 1: Collective Competence

Watch this video of Lorelei Lingard, PhD, talking about collective competence: https://www.youtube.com/watch?v=vI-hifp4u40.

DISCUSSION QUESTIONS

1. What are your first impressions of the information presented in the video?

2. Think about the teams you have worked on in the past. Do you think the team had collective competence? Why or why not?

3. Review Table 1.1. Why do we hold onto the myths described here? Have you seen examples of the truths in your experience working on teams? What was that experience like?

Activity 2: Learning About Heath Care Professional Roles and Teams

Identify someone from a different health profession (not a nurse) and interview them about their role and how they work in teams. Potential questions or prompts are the following:

- Describe your role as a professional.
- What is the typical education path for your profession?
- How does someone in your profession become certified or licensed?
- What is your role on the health care team? Who are the other members of your team?
- What do you like most about working on a team? What is the biggest challenge?

Create your own questions based on what else you would like to know. Write a brief summary of the interview. Review the website of the interviewee's professional organization (e.g., American Dental Association or American Physical Therapy Association); you could also review specialty professional organizations such as the Association of Oncology Social Work or the American College of Obstetricians and Gynecologists.

DISCUSSION QUESTIONS

1. How does the professional organization describe the profession?

2. Does the organization's website mention teamwork or interprofessional collaboration? If so, what how do they characterize it and their role on the team?

3. Is the information provided similar to different to the information you gathered in the interview? Why or why not?

Activity 3: Bias and Hierarchies in Health Care

Listen to *Care to Connect* podcast, episode 4: "How Are We Really Doing in IPE?" from the Centre for Advancing Collaborative Healthcare & Education (CACHE) at the University of Toronto: https://ipe.utoronto.ca/podcasts-ip-healthcare-series.

DISCUSSION QUESTIONS

1. What do you think about the idea of having a dual identity of being a nurse and being part of the interprofessional team?

2. Have you observed or experienced bias based on professional roles in health care? How might that impact the individual? The team? The patient?

3. What assumptions or stereotypes exist about the different health professions? How might these assumptions or stereotypes interfere with interprofessional collaboration and patient care?

4. Think back to your own experiences in the health care setting. Have you seen examples of when the hierarchy was detrimental to the team? How about examples of when the hierarchy was useful? What worked and what did not?

5. Have you seen examples of effective teams working without a strict hierarchy? What made these teams effective?

6. How does the isolation of different professions from one another enable bias and hierarchical structures in health care?

REFERENCES

Agency for Healthcare Research and Quality. (n.d.). *Section 2: Explanation of key concepts and tools.* https://www.ahrq.gov/teamstepps-program/curriculum/team/tools/index.html

American Association of Colleges of Nursing. (2021). *The essentials: Core competencies for professional nursing education.* https://www.aacnnursing.org/essentials/download-order

American Association of Colleges of Nursing. (2023). *Guiding principles for competency-based education and assessment.* https://www.aacnnursing.org/essentials/tool-kit/guides-and-talking-points

Armstead, C., Bierman, D., Bradshaw, P., Martin, T., & Wright, K. (2016). Groups vs. teams: Which one are you leading? *Nurse Leader, 14*(3), 179–182. https://doi.org/10.1016/j.mnl.2016.03.006

Bachynsky, N. (2020). Implications for policy: The Triple Aim, Quadruple Aim, and interprofessional collaboration. *Nursing Forum, 55*(1), 54–64. https://doi.org/10.1111/nuf.12382

Berwick, D. M., Nolan, T. W., & Whittington, J. (2008). The Triple Aim: Care, health, and cost. *Health Affairs, 27*(3), 759–769. https://doi.org/10.1377/hlthaff.27.3.759

Bodenheimer, T., & Sinsky, C. (2014). From Triple to Quadruple Aim: Care of the patient requires care of the provider. *Annals of Family Medicine, 12*(6), 573–576. https://doi.org/10.1370/afm.1713

Dow, A., Appelbaum, N., & DiazGranados, D. (2015). Leadership frameworks for interprofessional learning. In D. Forman, M. Jones, & J. Thistlethwaite (Eds.), *Leadership and collaboration: Further developments for interprofessional education* (pp. 13–28). Palgrave Macmillan. https://doi.org/10.1057/9781137432094_2

Essex, R., Kennedy, J., Miller, D., & Jameson, J. (2023). A scoping review exploring the impact and negotiation of hierarchy in healthcare organisations. *Nursing Inquiry*, e12571. https://doi.org/10.1111/nin.12571

Institute for Healthcare Improvement. (n.d.). *Triple Aim.* https://www.ihi.org:443/Topics/TripleAim/Pages/default.aspx

Interprofessional Education Collaborative. (2016). *Core competencies for interprofessional collaborative practice: 2016 update.* https://ipecollaborative.org/uploads/APTR-HPCTF_IPE_Crosswalk_2013.pdf

Itchhaporia, D. (2021). The evolution of the Quintuple Aim. *Journal of the American College of Cardiology, 78*(22), 2262–2264. https://doi.org/10.1016/j.jacc.2021.10.018

Lingard, L. (2016). Paradoxical truths and persistent myths: Reframing the team competence conversation. *Journal of Continuing Education in the Health Professions, 36*, S19. https://doi.org/10.1097/CEH.0000000000000078

Nelson, S., Tassone, M., & Hodges, B. D. (2014). *Creating the health care team of the future: The Toronto model for interprofessional education and practice.* ILR Press.

Northouse, P. G. (2022). *Leadership: Theory and practice* (9th ed.). SAGE.

Nundy, S., Cooper, L. A., & Mate, K. S. (2022). The Quintuple Aim for health care improvement: A new imperative to advance health equity. *JAMA, 327*(6), 521–522. https://doi.org/10.1001/jama.2021.25181

Seaton, J., Jones, A., Johnston, C., & Francis, K. (2021). Allied health professionals' perceptions of interprofessional collaboration in primary health care: An integrative review. *Journal of Interprofessional Care, 35*(2), 217–228. https://doi.org/10.1080/13561820.2020.1732311

Sollami, A., Caricati, L., & Sarli, L. (2015). Nurse–physician collaboration: A meta-analytical investigation of survey scores. *Journal of Interprofessional Care, 29*(3), 223–229. https://doi.org/10.3109/13561820.2014.955912

World Health Organization. (2010). *Framework for action on interprofessional education and collaborative practice.* http://www.who.int/hrh/resources/framework_action/en/

CREDIT

CHAPTER 2

Leadership Style

Georgia L. Narsavage, PhD, APRN, CNS-BC, FAAN, FNAP, ATSF, and
Catherine S. Koppelman, MSN, RN, R, NEA, CNO, Executive Coach

---

KEY AACN COMPETENCIES, SUB-COMPETENCIES, AND CONCEPTS

Domain 6: Interprofessional Partnerships

Competency 6.3 Use knowledge of nursing and other professions to address health care needs.

- *Entry-Level Sub-Competency 6.3a* Integrate the roles and responsibilities of health care professionals through interprofessional collaborative practice.
- *Advanced-Level Sub-Competency 6.3d* Direct interprofessional activities and initiatives.

Domain 9: Professionalism

Competency 9.5 Demonstrate the professional identity of nursing.

- *Entry-Level Sub-Competency 9.5e* Demonstrate emotional intelligence.
- *Advanced-Level Sub-Competency 9.5h* Identify opportunities to lead with moral courage to influence team decision-making.

Continued

Continued

Domain 10: Personal, Professional, and Leadership Development

Competency 10.3 Develop capacity for leadership.

- *Entry-Level Sub-Competency 10.3b* Formulate a personal leadership style.

- *Entry-Level Sub-Competency 10.3h* 10.3e Use appropriate resources when dealing with ambiguity.

- *Advanced-Level Sub-Competency 10.3k* Influence intentional change guided by leadership principles and theories.

- *Advanced-Level Sub-Competency 10.3n* Participate in the evaluation of other members of the care team.

- *Advanced-Level Sub-Competency 10.3p* Advocate for the promotion of social justice and eradication of structural racism and systematic inequity in nursing and society.

Concepts for Nursing Practice

- Communication
- Ethics
- Health Policy

KEY TERMS

Leadership

Leadership style

Professionalism

Professional identity

Power and influence

Emotional intelligence

Communication

Self-awareness

Collaboration

Self-management

Ethics

Social awareness

Advocacy

Relationship management

Health policy

INTRODUCTION: WHAT IS LEADERSHIP?

Being a leader and developing a leadership style is important to nurses in all roles and settings. One does not need to hold a formal leadership role to become a leader. Leadership has been described as a process whereby an individual influences a group of individuals to achieve a shared goal (Northouse, 2007). A nurse providing patient care according to professional standards, with patient/family engagement and respect for others, is practicing leadership clinically. A leader can influence members of the nursing teams to practice professionally and shape cultural norms of clinical excellence on a patient care unit. Nurses also provide care within interprofessional (IP) teams. Leadership skills are essential for all the professionals within IP teams. Nurses, practicing with clinical excellence, collaborate with other IP team members to positively impact team decisions and improve plans of care. In health care, the shared goal of nursing and IP teams is to do what best serves the patient, resulting in quality outcomes. The American Association of Colleges of Nursing (AACN, n.d.) maintains that nurse leaders are needed to bring order out of the existing tumultuous and disparate health care delivery system, not just at the bedside, but also in policy and research arenas (https://www.aacnnursing.org/5b-tool-kit/about-5b-tool-kit). Sfantou et al. (2017) examined the importance of leadership and leadership style in health care settings. They identified that strategic leadership by health care professionals is crucial in multiple health care settings, and that leadership styles were significantly correlated with quality care. Both patients and health care professionals have identified leadership as a core element for integrated quality care. In addition, empowering leadership is related to patient outcomes by promoting greater nursing expertise through better retention of nurses and continuity of staffing. Haller et al. (2022) found that leadership training for professional nurses improved their ability to create an engaging culture, and their understanding of how personal leadership styles supports collaborative practice and team effectiveness. By applying leadership principles and theories, a leader can influence how someone, or something develops, behaves, or thinks and be guided by skills, abilities, and values of leadership. A nursing leadership goal can be to work with individuals in a way that maximizes individual and collective strengths to achieve a desired goal of improving patient and health outcomes (Iachini et al., 2019).

As nursing has evolved, a key social construct has been recognition of nursing as a profession. *Professionalism* involves thinking, acting, and feeling in a manner consistent with the characteristics, values, and norms of the nursing profession (AACN, 2021). An individual's *professional identity* is the representation of self, achieved at stages over time, during which characteristics, values, and norms of the nursing profession are internalized, resulting in an individual thinking, acting, and feeling like a member of the profession (Cruess et al., 2014; Rasmussen, 2018). Professional roles for interprofessional teamwork require a shared acknowledgment of each participating member's roles and abilities. Without this acknowledgment, adverse outcomes may arise from a series of seemingly trivial errors that effective teamwork could have prevented. For example, the night shift nursing team on a patient care unit has consistently positive patient outcomes, thanks to their teamwork, championed by several seasoned nurses with strong relationships. Everyone is treated with respect and support. The day shift nursing team is known for having cliques constantly complaining about workload and low morale. The nurse manager consistently gets positive patient satisfaction feedback for the night shift staff and care and complaints for the day shift staff. Identifying an effective leadership style to address this could result in fewer adverse outcomes. Professionalism and professional identity are foundational to a nurse's confidence, necessary for leadership in practice.

Using the knowledge of one's own role and professional identity and the roles of other professions to appropriately assess and address the health care needs of the patients and populations served can facilitate higher quality and safer care (Core Competencies for Interprofessional Collaborative Practice [IPEC], 2016). One of the most common medical errors is an error in medication administration, such as giving a medication at a wrong dose or to a patient who has a known allergy. For example, the nurse caring for a new postoperative patient reviews the pain medication order and is concerned that the dose is too high. She calls the pharmacist, who concurs. The nurse then calls the physician and shares that information. The physician thanks her for catching this error. The order is canceled and a new one is created. A systematic approach with nurses, physicians, and pharmacists working as a team to consistently verify medications and validate patient uniqueness can greatly reduce such errors (Rodziewicz et al., 2022).

Growing as a leader includes developing a *leadership style*, which is the way people are directed and motivated by a leader to achieve goals (Al Khajeh, 2018). To formulate a personal leadership style, the individual designs a deliberate plan to adopt and develop the skills of a selected leadership style consistent with personal and professional goals. Leadership styles are related to leadership theories that explain the characteristics, qualities, and behaviors needed to lead (Al Khajeh, 2018). A leadership theory is based on research of what type of leaders' values/behaviors/actions get better results from followers in achieving goals and why. A leadership theory that stresses relating to others with respect, listening, understanding, and confidence in others is enacted through those behaviors. For example, two new graduates on the same unit have different nurse preceptors. One is very rigid about the way things get done and disparages the new nurse in front of others when performance is not exactly how the preceptor had taught. The other preceptor takes the time to explain rationales for using specific interventions and when the nurse has discretion. This preceptor gives positive feedback in a constructive way. The goal of both preceptors is to assure that the new graduate is competent and safe in practice, but the leadership styles are very different. One is practicing autocratic leadership theory, and the other is practicing a relational leadership theory.

The tree key leadership theories/styles that have been shown to positively affect patient outcomes are transformational leadership, authentic leadership, and collaborative/shared leadership (Cummings et al., 2018, 2021). Characteristics of these leadership styles can be found in the box below.

TABLE 2.1 **Leadership Styles**

Transformational Leadership
• innovative intellectual stimulation • individualized consideration with empathy and mentoring • idealized influence as a role model • inspirational motivation with a clear vision, optimism motivation, and inclusion (Collins et al., 2019)
Authentic Leadership
• self-awareness; understanding own strengths/motives • high moral standards and values, role model, transparency • resilient and optimistic; has self-efficacy • engagement with team for trust, commitment, and job satisfaction (Algeri et al., 2022)
Collaborative/Shared Leadership
• based on matrix of skills, capabilities, and team strengths • collective employees = leaders • vertical and horizontal communication flow • polycentric, synergistic organization (Orchard et al., 2017)

Transformational leadership is a relational style that focuses on people and relationships and maximizes the potential of followers through encouragement of innovation, creativity, and intellectual stimulation (Bass & Avolio, 1994; Cope & Murray, 2017; Collins et al., 2019). Transformational leaders can use intentional collaboration across professions and with care team members, patients, families, communities, and other stakeholders to promote innovation, optimize care, enhance the health care experience, and strengthen outcomes. For example, the in-patient Pediatric General Medicine team set a goal to better engage patients and families in care decisions by strengthening coordination of care. Team members were having a difficult time attending in-person daily rounds because of conflicting schedules. Parents were frustrated in not knowing when they could talk to the physicians. It took several thoughtful planning meetings with all team members and a parent representative to come up with a solution that involved all members committing to a set time for walking bedside rounds to facilitate families in attending or calling in. That solution was eventually adopted by all in-patient teams across the hospital.

Authentic leadership is a style that emphasizes leader insight, transparency, and congruence in actions and personal or expressed beliefs (Algeri et al., 2022). For example, an authentic leader might participate in the evaluation of other members of the care team by providing constructive feedback and recommendations for professional development goals They may also lead team members to examine their clinical practice and/or performance in the role based on observations, experiences, and objective outcomes.

Collaborative/shared leadership is a style that emerges from the distribution of leadership influence across multiple individuals assuming (and perhaps divesting themselves) of leadership roles over time in both formal and informal roles over time (Iachini et al., 2019; Orchard et al., 2017). Examples of professionals who could participate with a nurse leader to address health care needs using a collaborative leadership style include nurses at all levels, physicians, pharmacists, occupational and physical therapists, social workers, and others. A collaborative leadership style can be seen in developing a plan of care that involves encouraging and respecting input from nursing and other health care professionals. For example, in the 1st week, a new graduate advanced practice registered nurse (APRN) who formerly was an RN in the Surgical Intensive Care Unit (ICU) assumed the care of a new patient from the Post-Anesthesia Care Unit (PACU) following an aneurysm repair. The unit intensivist physician and many of the nurses were with a patient in full cardiac arrest on the unit and not available. The APRN received a bedside report but had no physician orders. The patient was agitated and moving around in the bed moaning. Their blood pressure (BP) was dropping, and heart rate was increased. "Is it pain," the APRN wonders, "or, of more concern, bleeding?" The assigned RN agreed with the APRN's reasoning and went to ask the surgeon for assistance. The APRN increased IV fluids and ordered two units of blood. The patient went directly back to the operating room, where the surgeon found that the surgical site was bleeding and thanked the APRN for such quick action based on clinical judgment. Collaboration saved the patient's life.

When facing ambiguity, a personal leadership style can help in seeking out appropriate individuals and identifying needed resources before acting, in order to check one's thinking, gain knowledge, or provide clarity and meaning and avoid confusion. Resources may include policies, code of ethics, standards, consultants, or other team members.

SCENARIO 1: ENTRY-LEVEL RN LEADERSHIP STYLE

You are a new graduate RN on a 24-bed surgical unit in a 250-bed community hospital. You are 6 months out from your 3-month orientation. You are very happy on this unit and feel good about your clinical practice skills. You also like the unit and staff. You rotate shifts and have gotten to know the staff well. Your preceptor was a nurse who had been on this unit for 3 years. The preceptor is well organized, proficient, and very knowledgeable. You learned so much with consistent feedback on your practice in a very respectful and reassuring manner; they are an excellent role model for you.

Today you are on the day shift, and your preceptor is the charge nurse. The unit is almost full, with many patients expected to be discharges and postoperative patients to be admitted. On top of that, the supervisor reassigned one of the nurses to float to other units, and an unlicensed assistive personnel (UAP, nurse aide) called in that they would be a few hours late. There are four RNs with each assigned to six patients. The charge nurse has asked for a float UAP and pulled you aside after morning report hand-off to tell you that it will be very busy but they know you can do it and will check in with you frequently.

You start off by checking with the UAP, who has 12 patients, on what is needed. The UAP feels that the case load is overwhelming, and they need help. You promise to help the UAP with patient turns and a few patients for bathing. You start by going through the labs and pending orders. Then you visit each patient and assess them. You "touch base" every 2 hours with the UAP. You have three pending discharges and a full order sets for all six patients just seen by the surgical residents; two patients are 2 days' postop and progressing well; one patient was transferred to the unit at 5:00 a.m. via the Emergency Department (ED) after emergency exploratory surgery and removal of a large colon mass resulting in a colostomy, a nasogastric tube (NG) to suction, wound drains, a urinary catheter, and IV fluids. Now you feel overwhelmed. You feel anxious that you can't do this or may forget things and make a mistake. What do you do now?

Discussion Questions

1. What are the goals for the RN in this situation? Drawing on an RN professional identity, list knowledge, skills, and values the RN could rely on to confidently manage the situation.
2. What leadership style would be effective in the situation? Explain your choice.
3. Identify actions/tactics that are possible for the RN to use.
4. What risks are associated with those tactics?
5. How can the risks be mitigated?
6. What resources will the RN need to request or consider in the plan?

SCENARIO 1: ADVANCED-LEVEL NURSE LEADERSHIP STYLE

You are a new graduate APRN with 5 years of experience as a nurse in acute inpatient care. You were offered a position in a very large employed primary care practice. You are the first APRN in the practice of six primary care providers (PCPs). Your direct boss is the head of the PCP group. Your compensation is less than you had hoped for and is tied to metrics that include quality measures, patient satisfaction, productivity, revenue per case/ cost per case, and readmissions/ED visits of your patients. Your orientation to the practice was minimal and entailed shadowing a physician for a day, using physicians as a resource for 2–3 weeks and feedback at the end of each day. You are not assigned a medical assistant (MA) even though all the physicians have one. After the 3 weeks of orientation, you are assigned to see new patients, complete the history and physicals, draft a plan, and then have the physician come in to take over the care. This continued for 2 months with feedback that was positive, and you passed orientation. You now see patients for their Medicare annual physicals, diabetic patients for education, and uncomplicated new patients. Your understanding is that you will be scheduled 16 patients a day, or eight patients for a 4-hour block. You are pleased with your progress and growing autonomy, even though the MAs and physicians are not very helpful or friendly. After 6 months you meet with the head of the group for a more formal evaluation. You are seeing six patients in a block session and are running late with no lunch. The head thinks you are spending too much time with the patients. Your diagnostics and lab tests are too extensive, so your cost per case is too high. Revenue is lower than expected, although quality and patient satisfaction metrics are very good. You have been given the next 6 months to improve revenue or the group will not be able to keep you. You need a plan.

Discussion Questions

1. What are the goal/s for the APRN? Drawing on APRN professional identity, list knowledge, skills, and values they can rely on to confidently achieve that goal(s).
2. What leadership style would be effective in the situation? Explain your choice.
3. Identify actions/tactics that are possible for the APRN to use.
4. What risks are associated with those tactics?
5. How can the risks be mitigated?
6. What resources will the APRN need to request or consider in the plan?

These scenarios are designed to assist you to recognize a leader's need to build relationships, reduce team stress, defuse conflict, and improve job satisfaction. One of the keys to leadership is being able to identify and regulate one's own emotions and understand the emotions the others (Prezerakos, 2018).

This is termed *emotional intelligence* (EI), which involves the ability to recognize our own feelings personally and professionally, and those of others, to motivate ourselves, and to handle our emotions well to have the best outcomes for ourselves and for our relationships (Goleman, 1998). Emotional intelligence competencies have four domains: self-awareness, self-management, social awareness, and relationship management (Boyatzis & McKee, 2006).

TABLE 2.2 **Emotional Intelligence Domains**

Domain	Definition
Self-awareness	Having the ability to understand your own feelings, possess an accurate self-assessment of your strengths/weaknesses, and showing self-confidence (Drigas & Papoutsi, 2018).
Example	A new graduate RN is in a patient room when the medical teaching team comes in for morning bedside rounds. None of the team members have washed their hands. The new graduate does not speak up, feels guilty, knowing it is for patient safety but is too intimated by the attending physician, residents, and medical students to speak.
Self-management	The ability to control feelings and reactions so as not to be driven by impulsive behaviors and feelings in situations with others (Drigas & Papoutsi, 2018).
Example	A new grad RN just completed orientation and is assigned a patient who will have a bedside procedure with the surgical team. The new graduate has never assisted with a procedure like this and is very anxious about doing it. The unit is very busy. The new graduate seeks out an experienced nurse who talks through the procedure set up and process. The new grad informs the surgeon that this a first-time experience with this procedure. The surgeon proceeds and uses this as an opportunity for teaching.
Social awareness	Involves a person's ability to consider the perspectives of others and apply that understanding to interactions with them (Mansel & Einion, 2019).

Domain	Definition
Example	The social worker and case manager of a mental health IP team frequently disagree on patient discharge plans. The APRN member is concerned about how the disagreements are affecting the group dynamics that interfere with collaboration.
Relationship management	Applies the other three areas of EI to enhance our ability to communicate clearly, maintain good relationships with others, connect with those from other backgrounds, work well in teams, and manage conflict (Goleman 1998., Boyatzis & McKee, 2006).
Example	The social worker of a mental health IP team seeks out the APRN member of the team for assistance in how to resolve the disagreements occurring with the team case manager on discharge planning. The APRN confirms the concern about that situation and the negative effect on team collaboration. They discuss options the social worker can use to approach the case manager and engage in discussion about how to improve their relationship. The APRN also offers to join the discussion to help. The social worker declines the offer, thanks the APRN for the assistance.

Emotional intelligence (EI) is an integral part of leadership. EI can be a strong asset in assuming leadership of an interprofessional team, recognizing that multiple professionals are capable of assuming effective leadership roles and shared leadership based on situational expertise requirements and a need to achieve a common goal.

Effective nurse leaders wisely use power and influence to affect change. Power is the potential ability of one person/group to influence other people or group to achieve goals and outcomes (Daft, 2016). Influence is to affect or change how someone or something develops, behaves, or thinks (Cambridge Dictionary, 2023). Collaboration focuses on working with individuals in a way that maximizes individual and collective strengths to achieve a shared goal (Iachini et al., 2019).

Power and influence within teams requires communication as well as collaboration. Communication is more than just sending and receiving information. Effective communication and effective leadership are key characteristics of a good leader and are closely intertwined (Branwart, 2020). Nurse leaders must be skilled communicators in numerous relationships with patients, families, and interprofessional teams at the point of care as well as at organizational levels, in communities and groups, and even on a global scale in order to achieve results through others.

Ethics describes what is expected in terms of right and correct and wrong or incorrect in terms of behavior. As health care professionals, nurses are held to ethical principles described in the American Nurses Association's (2015) code of ethics (*Guide to the Code of Ethics for Nurses With Interpretive Statements: Development, Interpretation, and Application,* 2nd Edition, 2015). All other professionals have similar ethical statements to guide practice. Ethics and ethical practice are essential aspects of patient care. The ethical principles that nurses apply in practice are the principles of justice (fairness), beneficence (doing right thing for patients), nonmaleficence (do no harm), accountability (responsibility for own actions), fidelity (staying true to principles), autonomy (patient self-determination), and veracity (truthfulness). Ethical leaders display positive behaviors through their words and actions.

Advocacy is another important role for a nurse leader in inter-professional teams. Advocacy includes patient self-determination in care delivery, the promotion of social justice, and eradication of structural racism and systematic inequity in nursing and society. Applying nursing's core values to support the recognition of economic and political conditions that produce health inequalities provides a step forward in achieving health care for all, from the individual patient level to the mega system level. Advocacy often involves changing health policy and redesigning health care systems.

Health policy is usually of two types. Regulatory health policies help standardize and control people and industries. Examples include standards of care, access to care, patient rights, and health information privacy. Allocative health policies provide money or power to certain groups, often by taking it from somewhere else. Effective leadership is needed at all levels of the system for policy implementation. In collaboration with other professionals, nurses can provide an essential and appropriate level of leadership needed to reshape health policy for patient care mandates, resources, structures, and health care systems.

SCENARIO 2: ENTRY-LEVEL RN ETHICAL DILEMMA

Pat is a new graduate practicing for about 8 months in a surgical ICU. She loves the unit and the specialty. Today one of the two patients assigned was recently transferred to the unit after a code white on a surgical unit. This patient is 90 years old and had surgery for colon cancer. It was a huge surgery. The patient's condition deteriorated 2 days postop. The surgical team, patient, and family agreed to a do not attempt to resuscitate (DNAR) order with no intubation and comfort care only.

The patient is on a rebreather oxygen mask in obvious respiratory distress and is now confused and agitated. Pat is concerned that the patient is suffering and needs medication intervention. The respiratory therapist agrees and recommends a morphine IV. The CRNA, after the postop assessment, concurs. It is July, and there are new residents (recently graduated physicians) and recently promoted chief residents on service. The surgical service is rounding on their patients, and Pat shares the joint concerns about the patient's labored breathing and the interprofessional care team's recommendation to give morphine to alleviate the distress. The chief tells Pat to get anesthesia to intubate the patient. Pat reminds the chief that the patient was made DNAR yesterday by the former chief upon request of the patient and the family. The chief still wants the family phone number to talk about intubation.

Scenario 2 depicts an ethical dilemma that demonstrates the need for professional identity, emotional intelligence, and leadership to advocate for the patient and family when there is a difference of opinion among health care providers.

Discussion Questions

1. What are the goals for the interprofessional (IP) team in this situation? Drawing on RN, respiratory therapist (RT), and certified registered nurse anesthetist (CRNA) professional identities, list knowledge, skills, and values they can rely on to confidently manage this ethical dilemma.
2. What leadership style would be effective in the situation? Explain your choice.
3. What EI competencies match that leadership style for this situation?
4. Identify actions/tactics that are possible for the team members to use.
5. What risks are associated with those tactics?
6. How can the risks be mitigated?
7. What resources will the IP team need to request or consider in the plan?

SCENARIO 2: ADVANCED-LEVEL NURSE ETHICAL DILEMMA

You are a seasoned oncology nurse practitioner (NP) on the oncology team employed by a comprehensive cancer center within a large tertiary care hospital system with four hospital physicians and 20 oncology NPs. The service covers 24 hours a day/7 days a week (24/7). The reputation of the cancer center is exceptional, with top national ratings and National Cancer Institute funding. The health care system has multiple hospitals and ambulatory sites for cancer and other specialties. The overall system needs to generate a better profit margin. To that end they have launched a system-wide VALUE Initiative (n.d.) to lower costs and maintain high quality of care. VALUE is a measurable ratio of health outcomes to cost. All services have been compared to peers in terms of cost and care outcomes. Teams have been formed working with finance and quality units to improve based on peer data–based comparisons.

The cancer center has many outcomes that are lower cost than the database, but there are opportunities to lower high costs such as long length of stay, readmission rates, and ED visits. The medical director of the cancer center will cochair the team to redesign care delivery to achieve lower cost while maintaining or exceeding current quality outcome. The system chief nursing officer (CNO) has asked you to colead the team. You and the medical director, an excellent and respected gynecologic oncologist, have a very good working relationship. In examining the data listed by physician, there is a lot of variability. By looking at high-cost providers, you learn that one of the physicians is the medical director, who, along with others, does not use palliative care with their patients for symptom management; hospice is ordered only when death is eminent. Late referrals create more patient suffering. This has been as a major issue and frustration for the team and the nursing staff who care for these patients.

Discussion Questions

1. What are your goals as an APRN coleading this IP team? Drawing on APRN professional identity, list knowledge, skills, and values they can confidently rely on to achieve the goals.
2. What leadership style would be effective in the situation? Explain your choice.

3. What EI competencies match that leadership style for the APRN to effectively influence in this situation to achieve those goals?
4. Identify related EI actions/behaviors for the APRN to use in the situation with the colead physician and then with the IP team.
5. What risks are associated with the actions/behaviors?
6. How can the risks be mitigated?
7. What resources will the APRN need to request or consider in the plan?

APPLICATION TO PRACTICE: HOW DO WE DEVELOP OUR CAPACITY FOR LEADERSHIP?

There are multiple areas on which to focus in developing a capacity for leadership. Overall, eight areas are commonly described skills found in good leaders (Jones-Schenk, 2018).

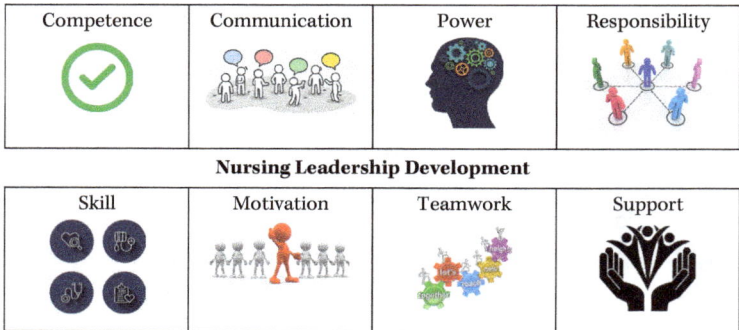

FIGURE 2.1 Common leadership skills.

How can you become a better leader? Although the exact steps you take will vary by your level of experience, personal characteristics, and your goals, three general steps can help you to be a leader.

Listen and learn. Leadership is about people skills, not power or control. The most successful leaders take time to listen and learn about their team members and their unique qualities they each have. Generate chances for your team members to make the most of their strengths and expand their effectiveness. Ask them for feedback and inquire about their perspectives. The more colleagues feel personally appreciated, the more you'll inspire them to work with enthusiasm toward goals that they personally care about.

Create collaborative goals. Leaders have a vision of where they want to go, and taking the time to learn about how team members' personal goals and visions could support the team goal helps everyone feel valued and involved in the overall greater mission. Discover your team members' core values and integrate them into larger team goals that advance the mission. Team members can then find more meaning and fulfillment and be motivated to be innovative in helping the team succeed.

Always seek ways to improve. Leaders look for every chance to better themselves and their teams. Get to know leaders you admire, and consider asking one of them to mentor you. Offer opportunities for open communication and feedback across all levels of your responsibility areas. When offering feedback, pair clear communication with additional resources for team members to develop their skills and expand their strengths. A leader supports the team in bringing their best to every situation, with creative feedback and continuous innovation.

Regardless of one's official position in a situation, leaders are known by their abilities to visualize, inspire, strategize, and support their teams toward goal attainment.

Why become a leader? Imagine effective nursing leadership practiced every day for every patient and family with compassion and excellence in a clinical environment that supports the nurse and the IP teams so that they can practice collaboratively the way it is "supposed" to be. Imagine the difference for patients, families, and care delivery. Imagine being passionate, appreciated, and satisfied knowing that what you do helps so many and enhances patient care, improves staff satisfaction, and supports you through the complex health care system. Without strong nurse leaders at the bedside to the boardrooms, we cannot achieve quality health care for all. You can have that in you own practice. Why? Because it is your choice how you practice. But it is not your choice how the systems work or how decisions are made in health care. Nurses at the point of care know better than anyone the challenges, policies, barriers, and inefficiencies of the health care systems but cannot change them. Nurses have ideas, solutions to problems, and innovations that can improve health care delivery, but they cannot make those decisions. So, your practice is impacted, and it is frustrating and drains your energy and satisfaction. Becoming a leader in your own practice is expected of all nurses in how they practice with professional values, standards, code of ethics, and respectful collaboration with other members of the IP teams. Aspiring to move beyond you own practice and be responsible for leadership of groups of patients, groups of professionals, programs of care, and so forth is the next level of leadership. Do you love to learn? Do you seek challenges? Do you want to make things better and take great pride in your work? You can do that in your own practice, but at some point in your career, consider moving beyond that. Your purpose extends to contributing and leading the change you want to see. It can start with a first step of leading a change on your unit, clinic, or group practice and grow over time to being a in a formal leadership position. Activity 1 at the end of this chapter walks you through the steps of creating your own leadership development plan.

DEVELOPING COLLABORATIVE LEADERSHIP SKILLS THROUGH INTERPROFESSIONAL EDUCATION

IPE is a valuable integrated component of health professional schools and related disciplines. Students in nursing, medicine, pharmacy, dentistry, and others, learning together about the concepts of health care and the provision of team-based health care services, have been able to improve patient-centered quality care and better provide safe care that can transform lives (IPEC, 2016). Students' perceptions of leadership have been changed as a result of inserting a collaborative leadership model, the social change model (SCM) of leadership, in an IPE course (Iachini et al., 2019). Essential elements of developing leadership skills include collaboration between health professional schools/faculty, respectful communication, reflection activities, application of knowledge and skills, and experience in interprofessional teams. The following activities and scenarios are designed to help you learn to lead through mentoring and understanding clinical ladder systems that are linked to interprofessional education.

Seeking a Mentor

Entry-level RN students in academia are assigned an advisor to guide them in their course of study. The same is true for graduate and doctoral nursing students. Other important roles in academia include professors, teachers, and clinical faculty. In clinical experiences, students will practice with preceptors who guide, clinically teach, and provide input into the evaluations on student competency. Students in doctoral programs, such as PhDs and DNPs, are assigned mentors who stay with students over the course of years of study to provide guidance and expertise in their professional development. All these roles influence the students in professional identity, knowledge, skills, and competence in their chosen career path. Upon graduation and following successful achievement of state boards and certifications, graduates enter practice, academia, or research. For new graduates to practice (RNs or APRNs), a preceptor in the clinical setting is assigned to orient them and confirm competency. Other roles new graduates will encounter regularly are peers, charge nurses, assistant nurse managers, nurse managers, shift supervisors, staff development instructors, nursing directors, and members of IP teams affiliated with the unit or setting. All these roles contribute to further influence the professional identity, knowledge, skills, and development of RNs and APRNs in practice settings. Nurses have so many opportunities to seek out a mentor among all these roles in academia and practice. So, what is a mentor? Why do you benefit from one? And how do you seek out one? To answer those questions, definitions of terms will be helpful.

A mentor is defined as an experienced person who advises and helps somebody with less experience over a period of time. A mentee is defined as a person who is advised and helped in their job by an experienced person over a period of time. Within the nursing profession, mentoring is described as a valued relationship and a nurturing process in which a more experienced person supports the professional growth and career development of another (Brunt & Bogdan, 2022; Hodgson & Scanlan, 2013). Like all relationships, the mentor–mentee relationship requires trust, effective communication, respect, and commitment to agreed-on purposes or shared goals. Mentoring is confidential, supportive, and respectful, leading to an ongoing relationship (Hodgson & Scanlan, 2013). Mentoring is so influential in one's career. The benefits are lifelong. One is fortunate to have such a relationship in which the mentor is committed to the mentee reaching their potential as a professional and in many cases a person.

That brings us to the third question: How do I seek a mentor? In practical terms, there are methods and means for a successful search for a mentor. Table 2.3 lists FAQS frequently raised about the mentoring process and suggestions on how to seek out a mentor. This table is also included in Activity 2 at the end of the chapter as a guide to help you identify a mentor. Consideration of a mentor is also strongly advised to provide real-time guidance and feedback on progress and to share their wisdom over time.

TABLE 2.3 **Seeking a Mentor**

FAQs	Entry-Level RN Suggestions	Advanced-Level Suggestions	My Plan
1) I am a new graduate. Would I benefit from having a mentor?	New graduate nurses will receive assistance and support in the transition to practice in the first year. A mentor at this time is not needed but relationships can be cultivated for the future. In the first year of practice as a novice nurse, there will be an orientation from 2–6 months with an experienced nurse preceptor depending on the specialty practice chosen. Many nurses connect with their preceptors and form a relationship that lasts past the orientation and can result in an informal mentor–mentee relationships that last for years. Other new nurses have close connections with the clinical instructors or professors from their education programs. They can reach out to them for advice and support in the transition to practice and stay connected over time as informal mentors. Many hospitals also have new nurse residency programs that offer monthly classes and support group programs with educators who assist with transition issues.	New graduate APRN nurses have orientations which differ in supports and length depending on the setting. Hospital based ARRNs typically are provided a longer structured orientation with assigned preceptors. Physician office setting may be shorter in orientation length and have less continuity with the same preceptor. For these reasons, a mentor is recommended to assist with the transition issues that APRNs face in the increased scope from the RN role and fewer supports. Seeking a mentor will be up to the APRN to secure and is confidential from the employer. Preceptors at clinical placement sites or professors from their training program can be a resource or can act as informal mentors.	

(Continued)

FAQs	Entry-Level RN Suggestions	Advanced-Level Suggestions	My Plan
2) How will I find a mentor?	There are many ways to seek a mentor. All the roles from academia and first year in practice experiences are all possibilities for a mentor. Nurses can be mindful of that possibility while in school and in practice. Look for RNs and APRNs that one admires and would aspire as role models. Move toward them in practice and get to know them. That is important to judge the fit and connect with them in their values and styles. Over time seek them out to check your thinking on clinical issues. Tell them how much you respect them and have learned from them. When you are clear that you would benefit from and want to commit to mentor-mentee relationship, ask them. Be prepared to share your development goal/s. Give them time to think it over and then follow up. Most nurses value mentoring other nurses. There are also nursing professional organization mentor programs and online programs for mentoring.	Seeking a mentor as a new APRN can begin in the educational program particularly at clinical placement sites. These clinicals provide the opportunity to have continuity with a preceptor/s for an entire semester at multiple sites over the length of the program. APRN faculty maintain a clinical practice and can be possible mentors as well. APRN students should be cultivating these relationships. Those who select positions in acute and ambulatory sites with other APRNs can connect with more seasoned APRNs as a resource and possible mentor. One can get to know the other and judge if they connect. It will be up to the new graduate APRN to move toward the seasoned APRN and discuss the possibility of a mentor-mentee relationship beyond the orientation period. Also, one can network with other new APRNs and faculty from the training program for possible referrals to seasoned APRNs. Search for online mentor programs by APRN specialty as well.	
3) Does a mentor charge a fee?	Typically, there is no charge for the informal mentor-mentee relationship. Be mindful of the mentor's time by following your plan and committing to the process. The online and professional organization programs require fees.	Typically, there is no charge for the informal mentor-mentee relationship. Be mindful of the mentor's time by following the plan and committing to the process. The online and professional organization programs require fees.	

FAQs	Entry-Level RN Suggestions	Advanced-Level Suggestions	My Plan
4) Does a mentor need to be a nurse?	Whether the mentor is a nursing professional or another type of professional will depend on the development goals. The mentor needs to have expertise and experiences in the developmental area to which the mentee aspires to grow professionally. Goals related to gaining more expertise in a nursing specialty, career counseling, considering a new position in nursing, and so on would require a nurse mentor. Goals that relate to leadership development could be from another profession such as organizational development, seasoned leaders in organizations or experts who teach leadership. One must weigh the connection with the mentor and the ability of the mentor to relate to the mentee's reality in making that choice.	Whether the mentor is a nursing professional or another type of professional will depend on the development goals. The mentor needs to have expertise and experiences in the developmental area to which the mentee aspires to grow professionally. Goals related to gaining expertise in a specialty would require a nurse mentor but could also be a physician in that specialty. Goals related to career counseling in nursing, seeking a new nursing role, and so on require a nurse mentor. Goals related to leadership development could involve a mentor from another profession such as organizational development, seasoned leaders in organizations or experts who teach leadership. One must weigh the connection with the mentor and the ability of the mentor to relate to the mentee's reality in making that choice.	
5) How long does a mentor work with you?	A mentor stays with the mentee over time. In the beginning of the relationship, the time together face to face or online will be more frequent and regular based on the plan and the progress toward the goals. When both parties agree the goals have been achieved, the relationship transitions into a touch base and as needed contact initiated by the mentee.	A mentor stays with the mentee over time. In the beginning of the relationship, the time together face to face or online will be more frequent and regular based on the plan and the progress toward the goals. When both parties agree the goals have been achieved, the relationship transitions into a touch base and as needed contact initiated by the mentee.	

Clinical Ladder

Mentoring is especially helpful within health care systems in that nursing departments provide a clinical ladder to encourage ongoing professional development. The clinical ladder is designed for an RN, and in some systems there are separate APRN clinical ladder programs. The overall goal is to motivate nurses to grow professionally and stay within the health care system. As a retention tool, the clinical ladder provides a pathway for ongoing development while remaining in a clinical RN or APRN position, with advancement in title, responsibilities, and salary. There is no standard ladder across nursing departments, but typically there are one to four levels. There are expectations that advance in each level, and leadership development expectations are often integrated. The criteria or competencies can relate to nursing care quality, ongoing education, nursing leadership, and other areas specific to the system, such as professional collaboration or interprofessional leadership expectations. Evaluation of meeting the level expectations will require the nurse to provide evidence of performance and achievement, peer review, and nurse manager review. Evaluation would involve a systematic determination and asaessment of the evidence for the nurse's merit, worth, and significance, using criteria consistent with the characteristics, values, and norms of the nursing profession and the health care system. Promotion and/or retention is determined by the annual evaluation and can result in a salary adjustment beyond the cost-of-living adjustment. (The following website demonstrates a clinical ladder and progression of levels: https://www.pennstatehealth.org/sites/default/files/2020-08/Domains-of-Practice-Descriptions.pdf.)

SCENARIO 3: ENTRY-LEVEL RN INTERPROFESSIONAL LEADERSHIP

The RN has practiced on a busy 40-bed medical/surgical unit in a large, urban inner city academic medical center and is committed to this patient population. Over the course of 6 years of practice the RN has completed her RN to BSN degree, became a charge nurse, a preceptor for new graduate orientees, and the unit Magnet champion representing the unit on the Nursing Central Shared Governance Coordinating Council. After becoming board certified in medical/surgical nursing, the nurse served on the unit-level quality committee and led many quality improvement initiatives on the unit; they are deeply respected and known for effective leadership, progressing from level 1 to the top level 4 of the nursing clinical ladder program. In that level, annual evaluations of nurses on the unit are completed as delegated by the nurse manager.

That last promotion was a result of assuming a patient care coordinator (PCC) position on the unit. This role is unit based in clinical practice, having knowledge about the plans of care and readiness for discharge of all the patients on the unit and representing nursing in daily interprofessional rounds. The PCC huddles with each nurse prior to and after rounds to get and give updates and assist with the plans of care. The consistent core IP rounding team members include the RN care coordinator, the social worker, and the RN case manager. Other members are not consistent people because they rotate who attends the rounds from within their respective departments. These members include a physical therapist, a pharmacist, a nutritionist, a resident physician from the teaching team, and a medical student. The last two members change frequently from week to week. The PCC, the social worker, and the RN case manager are very collaborative in their styles.

The team has adopted consistent processes, such as rotating the leader role weekly, adopting a standard format for patient presentation, and using an inclusive and respectful approach in seeking all member input. The team prioritizes patients for review based on long lengths of stay and frequency of readmissions, which can result in payment penalties or loss of revenue for the hospital. More importantly, these patients are complex and require thoughtful effective care planning for the patients' health and well-being. In today's meeting the top priority patient is a 30-year-old African American male patient with sickle cell disease since birth. He is frequently readmitted for pain episodes and is well known by the team. Plans of care are agreed on but infrequently followed by the patient postdischarge from the hospital. Written plans are posted in the electronic health record for all physicians on the service who may not be familiar with the patient.

Contracting with the patient to follow the plan has been tried and repeatedly fails. The medical student is new to the service and to the team. After introductions, the PCC presents the patient and the plan of care to date. The main concern is that morphine (a narcotic) is not easing the patient's pain. He is also very agitated with the nurses because they cannot give him any more pain medication than ordered and the medical student is very reluctant to raise the dose or frequency. The resident agrees with the medical student and wants the patient discharged. The medical team and the nursing staff have tried to work with this patient, but he in noncompliant. Many on the team have expressed concerns that the patient is "a frequent flyer and drug seeker." The PCC responds that they understand the team's frustrations but do not feel that characterization and labeling of the patient is appropriate given the nature of his disease. Other members of the team provide input. The pharmacist agrees with the medical team and shares that it is hard to believe that the patient has the degree of pain he reports because the dose is as high as they can give safely. The case manager shares that the patient is homeless and unemployed, so discharging him to the street will only result in him being readmitted through the ED. The social worker is openly distressed with the discussion and the biases expressed, which are offensive for any African American. The social worker believes that the proposed treatment is morally and ethically wrong. The group dynamic is now very tense, which uncharacteristic of this team. The PCC acknowledges that feelings of frustration and group member interaction are real and uncomfortable for the team and that they need to reflect on what this patient needs. A pain management specialist could be helpful. The social worker thinks an ethics consultant should be invited to help the team with their feelings. The case manager suggests inviting a member of the readmission team along with an outpatient case manager who could follow the patient after discharge and get him housing. The PCC works to schedule another meeting within a week. Together the IP team needs a thoughtful plan with the patient's involvement.

Discussion Questions

Put yourself in the position of the PCC nurse. Reflect on her leadership competencies, style, and development needs in clinical practice.

1. What is the immediate goal(s) for the PCC in practice right now? Discuss self-awareness and social awareness of these multiple responsibilities and how to manage the situation.
2. Characterize the PCC's professional identity. What knowledge, skills, and values would be helpful in managing the situation?
3. What EI competencies are needed in the situation? What leadership style encompass those competencies? Explain.
4. Identify IP actions/interventions that are possible for the PCC in the situation. What resources will be needed?
5. What risks are associated with those tactics?
6. How can the risks be mitigated?

SCENARIO 3: ADVANCED-LEVEL NURSE INTERPROFESSIONAL LEADERSHIP

You are a very seasoned CRNA working for a large anesthesia group that is contracted with a 600-bed community teaching hospital with a large surgical service. The hospital is an accountable care organization (ACO) for Medicare members and is in a Medicaid managed care state with a high rate of poverty. The group believes in shared governance, and all the members are represented in a governance council for major group decisions and plans. Members include anesthesiologists, you and another CRNA, anesthesia assistants, and the president and the chief financial officer of the group. Norms in the group among members are respect, teamwork, collaboration, and trust. You are seen as a leader, with effective working relationships with so many in the department regardless of role. You have precepted several new CRNAs and clinically mentored many. You are enthusiastic about patient safety and quality improvement and have experience in numerous improvement projects. One of your responsibility areas for the group is quality improvement responsibility for the group. You were mentored into the role by a seasoned anesthesiologist who recently retired. It has been fascinating to watch the group dynamics and to learn about rational decision-making and group processes. You have participated in major changes for the group already, such as new clinical policies/standards, selecting new equipment, updating the scheduling system, and implementing many quality improvement initiatives. A recent federal inspection found a serious deficiency for surgical, anesthesia, and nursing services in the operating rooms with inconsistent compliance to national patient safety goals. Without correction, the hospital could be denied payment for Medicare and Medicaid patients. You are asked to work with the Departments of Quality, Surgery, Anesthesia and Nursing to develop and implement a quality improvement plan within 2 weeks, and inspectors will visit again within 3 months for compliance.

Discussion Questions

Put yourself in the position of the APRN CRNA. What leadership style, knowledge, skills, values, and competencies would be most helpful to you?

1. What are the goals for the APRN/CRNA in this IP situation? Drawing on CRNA professional identity, list knowledge, skills, and values needed to confidently achieve those goal(s).
2. What leadership style do you use? Explain your choice.
3. What EI and leadership competencies match that leadership style for you to effectively influence the improvement plan and confidently achieve those goals?
4. What interprofessional competencies would be needed with this team?
5. Would you benefit from a mentor? How would you go about seeking a mentor given the timeline?
6. What tactics do you recommend? Identify risks associated with those tactics. How can they be mitigated?

CONCLUSION

Being a leader and developing a leadership style is important to nurses in all roles and settings. In health care, the shared goal of nursing and IP teams is to do what best serves the patient, resulting in quality outcomes. The AACN maintains that nurse leaders are needed to bring order out of the existing tumultuous and disparate health care delivery systems, not just at the bedside clinically, but also in policy, administration, and research arenas. Nursing professionalism is based on characteristics, values, and norms of the nursing profession creating a nurse's professional identity, which is foundational for nurse leaders.

Relational leadership styles have been significantly correlated with quality care and one's values, beliefs, and behaviors. When facing ambiguity, a personal leadership style can help in seeking out appropriate individuals and identifying needed resources before acting to check one's thinking, gain knowledge, or provide clarity and meaning and avoid confusion. A shared collaborative leadership style can be seen in developing a plan of care that involves encouraging and respecting input from nursing and other health care professionals. With IP teamwork, nurses can also move beyond their own practice and be responsible for leadership of groups of patients, groups of professionals, and programs of care. Interprofessional teamwork requires a shared acknowledgment of each participating member's roles and abilities. A systematic approach with teamwork of nurses, physicians, and other professionals can reduce errors. Examples of professionals that could participate with a nurse leader to address health care needs using a collaborative leadership style would be nurses at all levels, physicians, pharmacists, occupational and physical therapists, social workers, and others.

EI is an integral part of leadership. Effective communication and effective leadership are key characteristics of a good leader and are closely intertwined. Ethics, ethical practice, and advocacy are also essential aspects of patient care and integral to effective leadership. Mentoring is important in developing leadership skills, and especially helpful within health care systems where nursing departments provide clinical ladder programs to encourage ongoing professional development. Their overall goal is to motivate nurses to grow professionally and stay within the health care system. As a retention tool, the clinical ladder provides a pathway for ongoing development while remaining in a clinical

RN or APRN position, with advancement in title, responsibilities, and salary. In this chapter we identified the AACN competencies that pertain to nursing leadership, provided background on developing leadership skills, explained why leadership is important for nurses, and identified individual and system-level strategies that help nurses become effective leaders. We also included advanced-level sub-competencies pertaining to leadership. Nurses can also implement competencies from other domains, and we included learning activities to apply the content.

KEY POINTS

- Professionalism and professional identity are foundational to leadership in practice.
- To develop a leadership style, individuals design a plan to adopt and develop the competencies of a selected leadership style consistent with personal and professional goals.
- Leadership theories are based on research of what type of values/behaviors/actions by leaders influence others and get better results from followers.
- Important details in this chapter are three general steps to becoming a better leader: listening and learning, creating collaborative goals, and seeking ways to improve.
- Nurses can become leaders in their own practice by following professional values, standards, code of ethics, and respectful collaboration with other members of the IP teams.
- Effective nurse leaders wisely use power and influence to effect positive change.

ACTIVITIES

Activity 1: Making a Leadership Development Plan

The tools that follow are designed to guide you in your leadership development journey and process. Self-assessment is beneficial in learning new skill sets that will help you become a leader (Dubrin, 1988; Institute for Health and Human Potential, n.d.; Mind Tools Content Team, n.d.). The following assessments may be useful to you, and are easily accessible:

The Leadership Motivation Assessment MindTools: https://www.mindtools.com/acty452/the-leadership-motivation-assessment content team; patterned after A.J. DuBrin (1998) *MindTools Leadership Skills Assessment in Leadership: Research Findings, Practice and Skills* (2nd edition). Use the following template to create your individual leadership development plan. Additional resources are listed in another table for easy reference.

Name: _____ Individual Leadership Development Plan			
Action	**Timeline**	**Resources**	**Outcome Metric/ Status**
1. Reflect on and define your personal and professional values.			
2. Complete a self-assessment of your leadership strengths and areas that need further development. Ask for feedback from peers, role models, and trusted colleagues about their perceptions.			
3. List these areas as competencies.			
4. Increase your knowledge and learning of leadership styles.			
5. Compare your values and leadership strengths with the leadership styles and related competencies.			
6. Choose a leadership style that matches your values and includes some of your strengths as well as competencies you need to development.			
7. Start practicing new competencies. Keep a journal and reflect on those practice experiences.			
8. Seek out a mentor to guide you over time in your growth as a leader.			

Career Ladder Resources

Resource	Description	Source
AACN (American Association of Colleges of Nursing)	Transform academic leadership with leadership development programs for faculty and deans, a diversity leadership institute, mentor links, and leadership networks.	https://www. aacnnursing.org/ conferences-webinars/ leadership-development
AONL (American Association for Nursing Leadership)	Nursing leadership programs: 6-month virtual leadership lab for nurse managers; Virtual Nurse Manager Institute 3-day intensive program; executive leadership programs.	https://www.aonl. org
Attributes of a Successful Clinical Ladder program	Professional development and advancement career ladder for nurses. Includes leadership demonstration in practice. Designed to keep nurses at point-of-care delivery.	https://pubmed. ncbi.nlm.nih. gov/31149778/ Requires permission of author to copy any materials
Becoming a Resonate Leader	Book written by Annie McKee, Richard Boyatzis, and Frances Johnston on how to become a resonate leader. Book details reflections, self-assessments, and a learning contract for intentional change. This leadership style is like other relational leadership styles.	McKee, A., Boyatzis, R. E., & Johnston, F. (2008). Becoming a resonant leader. Harvard Business Review Press.

Activity 2: Seeking a Mentor

Another step in developing as a leader is finding a mentor to help you grow in your career. Review the FAQs and suggestions in the table and create a plan to help you identify a mentor.

FAQs	Entry-Level RN Suggestions	Advanced-Level Suggestions	My Plan
1) I am a new graduate. Would I benefit from having a mentor?	New graduate nurses will receive assistance and support in the transition to practice in the first year. A mentor at this time is not needed but relationships can be cultivated for the future. In the first year of practice as a novice nurse, there will be an orientation from 2–6 months with an experienced nurse preceptor depending on the specialty practice chosen. Many nurses connect with their preceptors and form a relationship that lasts past the orientation and can result in an informal mentor–mentee relationships that last for years. Other new nurses have close connections with the clinical instructors or professors from their education programs. They can reach out to them for advice and support in the transition to practice and stay connected over time as informal mentors. Many hospitals also have new nurse residency programs that offer monthly classes and support group programs with educators who assist with transition issues.	New graduate APRN nurses have orientations which differ in supports and length depending on the setting. Hospital based ARRNs typically are provided a longer structured orientation with assigned preceptors. Physician office setting may be shorter in orientation length and have less continuity with the same preceptor. For these reasons, a mentor is recommended to assist with the transition issues that APRNs face in the increased scope from the RN role and fewer supports. Seeking a mentor will be up to the APRN to secure and is confidential from the employer. Preceptors at clinical placement sites or professors from their training program can be a resource or can act as informal mentors.	

(Continued)

FAQs	Entry-Level RN Suggestions	Advanced-Level Suggestions	My Plan
2) How will I find a mentor?	There are many ways to seek a mentor. All the roles from academia and first year in practice experiences are all possibilities for a mentor. Nurses can be mindful of that possibility while in school and in practice. Look for RNs and APRNs that one admires and would aspire as role models. Move toward them in practice and get to know them. That is important to judge the fit and connect with them in their values and styles. Over time seek them out to check your thinking on clinical issues. Tell them how much you respect them and have learned from them. When you are clear that you would benefit from and want to commit to mentor-mentee relationship, ask them. Be prepared to share your development goal/s. Give them time to think it over and then follow up. Most nurses value mentoring other nurses. There are also nursing professional organization mentor programs and online programs for mentoring.	Seeking a mentor as a new APRN can begin in the educational program particularly at clinical placement sites. These clinicals provide the opportunity to have continuity with a preceptor/s for an entire semester at multiple sites over the length of the program. APRN faculty maintain a clinical practice and can be possible mentors as well. APRN students should be cultivating these relationships. Those who select positions in acute and ambulatory sites with other APRNs can connect with more seasoned APRNs as a resource and possible mentor. One can get to know the other and judge if they connect. It will be up to the new graduate APRN to move toward the seasoned APRN and discuss the possibility of a mentor-mentee relationship beyond the orientation period. Also, one can network with other new APRNs and faculty from the training program for possible referrals to seasoned APRNs. Search for online mentor programs by APRN specialty as well.	
3) Does a mentor charge a fee?	Typically, there is no charge for the informal mentor-mentee relationship. Be mindful of the mentor's time by following your plan and committing to the process. The online and professional organization programs require fees.	Typically, there is no charge for the informal mentor-mentee relationship. Be mindful of the mentor's time by following the plan and committing to the process. The online and professional organization programs require fees.	

FAQs	Entry-Level RN Suggestions	Advanced-Level Suggestions	My Plan
4) Does a mentor need to be a nurse?	Whether the mentor is a nursing professional, or another type of professional will depend on the development goals. The mentor needs to have expertise and experiences in the developmental area to which the mentee aspires to grow professionally. Goals related to gaining more expertise in a nursing specialty, career counseling, considering a new position in nursing, etc. would require a nurse mentor. Goals that relate to leadership development could be from another profession such as organizational development, seasoned leaders in organizations or experts who teach leadership. One must weigh the connection with the mentor and the ability of the mentor to relate to the mentee's reality in making that choice.	Whether the mentor is a nursing professional, or another type of professional will depend on the development goals. The mentor needs to have expertise and experiences in the developmental area to which the mentee aspires to grow professionally. Goals related to gaining expertise in a specialty would require a nurse mentor but could also be a physician in that specialty. Goals related to career counseling in nursing, seeking a new nursing role etc, require a nurse mentor. Goals related to leadership development could involve a mentor from another profession such as organizational development, seasoned leaders in organizations or experts who teach leadership. One must weigh the connection with the mentor and the ability of the mentor to relate to the mentee's reality in making that choice.	
5) How long does a mentor work with you?	A mentor stays with the mentee over time. In the beginning of the relationship, the time together face to face or online will be more frequent and regular based on the plan and the progress toward the goals. When both parties agree the goals have been achieved, the relationship transitions into a touch base and as needed contact initiated by the mentee.	A mentor stays with the mentee over time. In the beginning of the relationship, the time together face to face or online will be more frequent and regular based on the plan and the progress toward the goals. When both parties agree the goals have been achieved, the relationship transitions into a touch base and as needed contact initiated by the mentee.	

REFERENCES

Al Khajeh, E. H. (2018). Impact of leadership styles on organizational performance. *Journal of Human Resources Management Research,*.

Algeri, E. D. B. O., Silveira, R. S. D., Barlem, J. G. T., Costa, M. C. M. D. R., Stigger, D. A. D. S., & Dan, C. S. (2022). Authentic leadership in nurses' professional practice: An integrative review. *Rev Bras Enferm.*, *75*(1), e20210972. https://doi.org/10.1590/0034-7167-2021-0972

American Association of Colleges of Nursing. (n.d.). *5B tool kit.* https://www.aacnnursing.org/5b-tool-kit

American Association of Colleges of Nursing. (2021). *The essentials: Core competencies for professional nursing education.* https://www.aacnnursing.org/Essentials

Bass, B. M., & Avolio, B. J. (Eds.) (1994). *Improving organizational effectiveness through transformational leadership.* SAGE.

Boyatzis, R. E., & McKee, A. (2006) Intentional change. *Journal of Organizational Excellence*, *25*(3), 49–60. https://doi.org/10.1002/joe.20100

Branwart, M., (2020) Communication studies: Effective communication leads to effective leadership, *New Directions for Student Leadership, 3*(165) 87–97.

Brunt, B. A., & Bogdan, B. A. (2022). *Nursing professional development leadership.* StatPearls. https://www.ncbi.nlm.nih.gov/books/NBK519064/

Cambridge Dictionary (2023) B2. https://dictionary.cambridge.org/us/dictionary/english/influence?q=INFLUENCE

Collins, E., Owen, P., Digan, J., & Dunn, F. (2019). Applying transformational leadership in nursing practice. *Nursing Standard*, *35*(5), 59–66. https://doi.org/10.7748/ns.2019.e11408

Cope, V., & Murray, M. (2017). Leadership styles in nursing. *Nursing Standard*, *31*(43), 61–70. https://doi.org/10.7748/ns.2017.e10836

Cruess, R. L., Cruess, S. R., Boudreau, J. D., Snell, L., & Steinert, Y. (2014). Reframing medical education to support professional identity formation. *Academic Medicine.*, *89*, 1446–1451.

Cummings, G. G., Lee, S., Tate, K., Penconek, T., Micaroni, S. P. M., Paananen, T., & Chatterjee, G. E. (2021). The essentials of nursing leadership: A systematic review of factors and educational interventions influencing nursing leadership. *International Journal of Nursing Studies.*, *115*, 103842. https://doi.org/10.1016/j.ijnurstu.2020.103842

Cummings, G. G., Tate, K., Lee, S., Wong, C. A., Paananen, T., Micaroni, S. P. M., & Chatterjee, G. E. (2018). Leadership styles and outcome patterns for the nursing workforce and work environment: A systematic review. *International Journal of Nursing Studies*, *85*, 19–60. https://doi.org/10.1016/j.ijnurstu.2018.04.016

Daft, Richard L. (2016). *Management*. Southwestern Cengage Learning, ISBN1285871839

Drigas, A.S., & Papoutsi, C. A. (2018). New layered model on emotional intelligence. *Behavioral. Science.*, 8, 45. https://doi.org/10.3390/bs8050045

DuBrin, A. J. (1998). *Leadership skills assessment in leadership: Research findings, practice and skills* (2nd ed.). Houghton Mifflin.

Goleman, D. (1998). The emotional intelligence of leaders. *Leader to Leader Issue*, *10*, 20–26. https://onlinelibrary.wiley.com/doi/10.1002/ltl.40619981008

Goleman, D., Boyatzis, R., & McKee, A. (2002). *Primal leadership: Realizing the importance of emotional intelligence*. Harvard Business School Press. https://psycnet.apa.org/record/2002-00650-000

Haller, A., Beck, D., Farkas, D., Murphy, E., Bartow, A., Meholic, D., Poerschke, R., & Massey, S. (2022). Outcomes of leadership training for PAs and NPs. *JAAPA*, *35*(12), 1. https://doi.org/10.1097/01.JAA.0000892816.07115.b2

Hodgson, A., & Scanlan, J. (2013) A concept analysis of mentoring in nursing leadership. *Open Journal of Nursing*, *3*, 389–394. https://doi.org/10.4236/ojn.2013.35052

Iachini, A. I., Dana, D., DeHart, T. B., Dunn, B. L., Blake, E. L., & Blake, C. (2019) Examining collaborative leadership through interprofessional education: Findings from a mixed methods study. *Journal of Interprofessional Care*, *33*(2), 235–242. https://doi.org/10.1080/13561820.2018.1516635

Institute for Health and Human Potential. (n.d.). Test your emotional intelligence. https://www.ihhp.com/free-eq-quiz/

Interprofessional Education Collaborative. (2016). *Core competencies for interprofessional collaborative practice: 2016 update.*

Jones-Schenk, J. (2018). National education progression in nursing (NEPIN). *JONA: The Journal of Nursing Administration*, *48*(11), 535–537. https://doi.org/10.1097/NNA.0000000000000674

Mansel, B., & Einion, A. (2019). "It's the relationship you develop with them": Emotional intelligence in nurse leadership. A qualitative study. *British Journal of Nursing*, *28*(21), 1400–1408. https://doi.org/10.12968/bjon.2019.28.21.1400

Mind Tools Content Team. (n.d.). *The leadership motivation assessment.* https://www.mindtools.com/acty452/the-leadership-motivation-assessment

Northouse, P. G. (2021). *Leadership theory and practice* (9th ed.). SAGE.

Orchard, C. A., Sonibare, O., Morse, A., Collins, J., & Al-Hamad, A. (2017). Collaborative leadership, part 1: The nurse leader's role within interprofessional teams. *Nursing Leadership*, *30*(2), 14–25. https://doi.org/10.12927/cjnl.2017.25258

Prezerakos, P. E. (2018). Nurse managers' emotional intelligence and effective leadership: A review of the current evidence. *Open Nursing Joournal., 12,* 86–92. https://doi.org/10.2174/1874434601812010086

Rasmussen, P., Henderson, A., Andrew, N., & Conroy, T. (2018). Factors influencing registered nurses' perceptions of their professional identity: An integrative literature review. *Journal of Continuing Education in Nursing., 49*(5), 225–232. https://doi.org/10.3928/00220124-20180417-08

Rodziewicz, T. L., Houseman, B., & Hipskind, J. E. (2022). *Medical error reduction and prevention.* StatPearls. https://www.ncbi.nlm.nih.gov/books/NBK499956/

Sfantou, D. F., Laliotis, A., Patelarou, A. E., Sifaki-Pistolla, D., Matalliotakis, M., & Patelarou, E. (2017). Importance of leadership style towards quality of care measures in healthcare settings: A systematic review. *Healthcare, 5*(4), 73. https://doi.org/10.3390/healthcare5040073

The Value Initiative. (2020). *Home page.* https://valueinitiative.com/

CREDITS

CHAPTER 3

Communication

Rita Sfiligoj, DNP, MPA, RN, Shannon Wong, MSN, RN, CPNP, Jesse Honsky, DNP, MPH, RN, PHNA-BC, and Carol Savrin, DNP, RN, CPNP, R, FNP-BC, FAANP, FNAP

KEY AACN COMPETENCIES, SUB-COMPETENCIES, AND CONCEPTS

Domain 2: Person-Centered Care

Competency 2.2 Communicate effectively with individuals.

- ***Entry-Level Sub-Competency 2.2c*** Use a variety of communication modes appropriate for the context.
- ***Advanced-Level Sub-Competency 2.2g*** Demonstrate advanced communication skills and techniques using a variety of modalities with diverse audiences.

Domain 6: Interprofessional Partnerships

Competency 6.1 Communicate in a manner that facilitates a partnership approach to quality care delivery.

- ***Entry-Level Sub-Competency 6.1b*** Use various communication tools and techniques effectively.
- ***Advanced-Level Sub-Competency 6.1.g*** Evaluate effectiveness of interprofessional communication tools and techniques to support and improve efficacy of team-based interactions.

Continued

Continued

Domain 8: Informatics and Health Care Technologies

Competency 8.1 Describe the various information and communication technology tools used in the care of patients, communities, and populations.

- *   ***Entry-Level Sub-Competency 8.1c*** Effectively use electronic communication tools.

Concepts for Nursing Practice

- • Communication
- • Compassionate care
- • Diversity, equity, and inclusion
- • Social determinants of health

KEY TERMS

Verbal communication
Nonverbal communication
Interprofessional communication

Intraprofessional communication
Interpersonal communication
Task communication

INTRODUCTION: WHAT IS COMMUNICATION?

Communication is how humans make sense of the world around them. Communication occurs as an interactive two-way process or interaction involving two or more people, such as verbal exchanges, writing, behaviors, body language, touch, and emotion (American Association of Colleges of Nursing [AACN], 2021). Effective communication occurs when the sender of a message shares the meaning of the message in a way that conveys the full intent of the message. As a result, the receiver of the message understands the intended information (Werder, 2019). Communication is a reciprocal process. In the health care literature, communication and interaction are often used interchangeably and describe the process of social and informational exchange between a sender and a receiver. The experience and skill of the people engaged in the interaction and the context in which the interaction occurs may impact the quality of communication (van Manen et al., 2021).

Communication failures between interprofessional team members are the most common cause of errors and adverse events in health care (Newell & Jordan, 2015). Communication affects patient satisfaction and is directly related to patient adherence to treatment. It has a direct impact on health outcomes and patient trust. Quality health care depends on communication exchanges between health care professionals and between the professionals and patients. Dahlke et al. (2020) identified that the communication processes needed to be improved to support interprofessional collaboration. Interprofessional collaboration requires clear communication to prevent duplicated or conflicting patient care and reduces clinical errors. This chapter explores concepts and skills for nurses to use when communicating with other health care professionals and patients.

Verbal Communication

Verbal communication is the process of conveying a message through spoken or written words (Crowe, 2017). Typical forms of verbal communication in health care include conversations held in person, over the phone, or by video call among health care professionals and patients. Common written formats include secure text or messaging applications, the EHR, and patient education materials. Important elements of verbal communication include using an appropriate vocabulary for the situation, speaking slowly and clearly, using an appropriate tone of voice, being brief and direct to avoid confusion, and providing information in a timely manner (Crowe, 2017).

Nonverbal Communication

Nonverbal communication relates to how a person communicates with their body instead of the exact words they speak or write (Sibiya, 2018). Like verbal communication, the exchange of nonverbal information involves whom you communicate with and how you communicate. Nonverbal clues can express the level of engagement during an interaction. Facial expressions, eye contact, body posture, physical distance, interaction with technology, and touch are all forms of nonverbal communication that express meaning. For example, smiling can express an attitude of caring behavior (Thakur & Sharma, 2021). If a health care professional or patient is preoccupied with an electronic device screen, others may perceive it as disinterest. Touching, such as placing a hand on a shoulder, is a nonverbal communication that may convey empathy and compassion. However, it is important to remember that not all people perceive nonverbal communication in the same way. For example, in some cultures, direct eye contact is perceived as an indication of attentiveness and interest. There are cultures, however, in which eye contact may be perceived as disrespectful, so it is avoided (Purnell, 2018). When interpreting nonverbal communication, health care professionals should remember that their perceptions of the behavior may differ from those of the other person or people involved in the interaction, so it is important to gain a better understanding of the situation by following up with questions and additional information before jumping to conclusions.

Task Communication

Task communication is a form of communication that focuses on the interactions between team members that help the team reach their common goals. This includes listening to each other, engaging in dialogue, sharing appropriate information, and making decisions collaboratively. More information and examples of task communication are available in Chapter 9.

Interpersonal Communication

Interpersonal communication refers to how individuals on a team communicate with each other. Teams with strong interpersonal communication skills feel psychologically safe, give and receive feedback respectfully, and positively manage conflict. More information and examples of interpersonal communication and conflict management are available in Chapter 8 and Chapter 9.

Discussion Questions

Review the definitions of the behaviors related to task communication and interpersonal communication in Chapter 9. After reading, answer the following questions:

1. What does respectful communication sound or look like to you? Include examples of both verbal and nonverbal communication.
2. Think about a time when you experienced or observed poor communication. What stands out to you about that situation? What were the consequences or outcomes of the situation?
3. How might engaging in dialogue, sharing appropriate information, and making decisions collaboratively facilitate task communication among team members? If those behaviors are lacking on a team, how might that impact patient care?
4. How might psychological safety on a team impact interpersonal communication, specifically their ability to give or receive feedback? How might it impact conflict management on a team?

APPLICATION TO PRACTICE: COMMUNICATION TOOLS FOR THE INTERPROFESSIONAL TEAM

Communication is essential to safe, quality patient care. It occurs almost constantly in our daily lives and health care settings. Take, for example, Mariana. Mariana is a nurse midwife in a busy clinic. On a typical day, she will greet the staff at the front desk with a smile and a wave as she enters the building in the morning, then steps into her office to review her email and secure messages. After filling a cup of coffee, she walks to the clinic and meets with the team, which includes a physician, medical assistant, pharmacist, and social worker. Before they start talking about the plan for the day, they take a little time to check in to see how everyone is doing. After the team agrees on the plan, they begin to see patients. Mariana then knocks on the exam room door and warmly greets the patient and their partner. She sits down, facing the couple, before she starts asking questions. When the appointment concludes, she documents it in the electronic health record (EHR). Later in the afternoon, the pharmacist calls Mariana and asks her about the prescription she wrote earlier in the morning; the dosage differed from what is normally prescribed. Mariana returned to the EHR and identified this as an error. She changed the prescription to the correct dose and thanked the pharmacist for bringing it to her attention.

In this scenario, there are examples of how communication facilitates safe and efficient care and helps Mariana connect interpersonally with her patients and team members. Since communication is so important to health care, many tools and strategies have been developed to help the interprofessional team communicate effectively. This section will discuss some of those tools and how they can be used in health care.

TeamSTEPPS® 3.0 Framework

The Strategies and Tools to Enhance Performance and Patient Safety (TeamSTEPPS®) is an evidence-based teamwork approach that aims to improve communication among health care professionals and provide safe and high-quality patient outcomes. The framework includes a curriculum for training interprofessional teams and can be used in all areas of health care.

The Agency for Healthcare Research and Quality (AHRQ) and the Department of Defense (DoD) developed the program as part of the government's response to improve patient safety (Parker et al., 2019). In 2023, TeamSTEPPS 3.0 was introduced with updates to the framework and tools to facilitate team communication. The key skills in TeamSTEPPS® 3.0 framework are communication, team leadership, situation monitoring, and mutual support (AHRQ, 2023a see Figure 3.1 and Table 3.1).

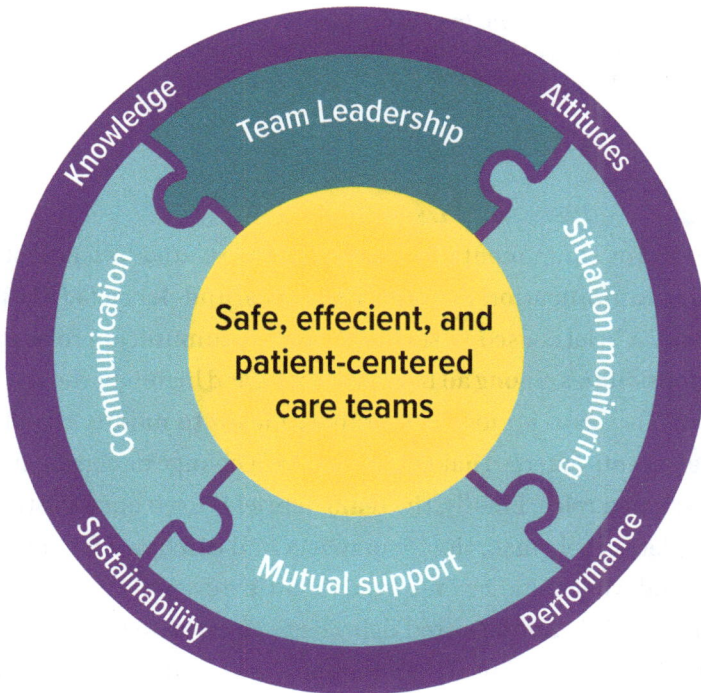

FIGURE 3.1   TeamSTEPPS® 3.0 framework and competencies.

TABLE 3.1   **TeamSTEPPS® 3.0 Key Skills and Definitions**

Communication	A verbal and nonverbal process by which information can be clearly and accurately exchanged among team members.
Team leadership	Ability to lead teams to maximize the effectiveness of team members by ensuring that team actions are understood, changes in information are shared, and team members have the necessary resources.
Situation monitoring	Process of actively scanning and assessing situational elements to gain information or understanding or to maintain awareness to support team functioning.
Mutual support	Ability to anticipate and support team members' needs through accurate knowledge about their responsibilities and workload.

Note. Retrieved from the TeamSTEPPS® 3.0 pocket guide, n.d., https://www.ahrq.gov/teamstepps-program/resources/pocket-guide/index.html.

Briefs, Huddles, and Debriefs

Important components in TeamSTEPPS® related to leadership and communication are briefs, huddles, and debriefs (AHRQ, 2023a). A brief is used to share the plan, communicate roles and responsibilities among all team members, and highlight the team's goals. The team huddle is a strategy meant to modify the plan when events emerge that might require a change or clarification in assigned roles. Finally, the team debrief is used once the team completes their task; the team meets and discusses what went well and what could be improved for future events. Team leaders can use briefs, huddles, and debriefs to help the team come to a shared understanding of the situation, tasks, and responsibilities, also called a shared mental model (AHRQ, 2023a).

Closed Loop Communication

Closed-loop communication (see Figure 3.2) is the verbal process in which the sender and receiver of the message confirm that the information provided is understood by everyone involved using the methods of call-out, check-backs, and teach-back (AHRQ, 2023b). Call-out is typically used in urgent or emergency situations. It is used to give information to all team members simultaneously, help the team anticipate what to do next, and name the individual responsible for carrying out the task. It can be adapted to nonurgent situations as needed. Check-back is a process in which the receiver of the message confirms understanding of the information sent by the sender.

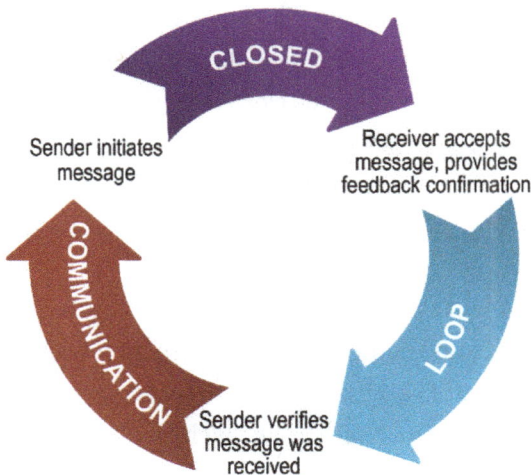

FIGURE 3.2   Closed-loop communication.

Example Call-Out

Ming walks into Mr. Jones's exam room in the clinic and finds him unresponsive. Ming pushes the code blue button in the room, calls out into the hallway, and says, "Mr. Jones in room

205 is unresponsive. I need help here. Drew, bring the crash cart down here immediately."

Example of Check-Back

Regina: "Brian, the orders for Ms. Rodriguez were updated this morning. Please check her blood sugar before she eats her lunch today."

Brian: "Yes, I will check Ms. Rodriguez's blood sugar today before she eats her lunch.

Regina: "Correct, thank you."

Discussion Questions

1. How have you used closed-loop communication in the clinical setting or your daily life?
2. Think of a situation when close-loop communication would be helpful. What would you say in that situation, as the sender or receiver of the message?

Teach-back is a method of communication frequently used with patients and their caregivers to assess if they have a clear understanding of the information shared with them (AHRQ, 2023b). More information about teach-back is in this chapter's Communication With Patients section.

Handoff

A handoff in health care occurs when information, authority, and responsibility are transferred. An effective handoff includes a transfer of responsibility and accountability, clarity of information, verbal communication of information, acknowledgment by the receiver, and an opportunity to review the situation with a "new pair of eyes" (AHRQ, 2023b). An opportunity to ask questions and clarify and confirm patient conditions is part of an effective handoff to ensure patient safety. These transitions often occur in shift changes when there is a transfer of responsibility between and among health care professionals. It also occurs when transferring a patient to a different floor or environment for a test or procedure. During a formal handoff, a health care professional or team passes responsibility and accountability to another. Therefore, it is essential to determine and accept who is responsible for patient care and decision-making during the handoff.

Inadequate communication or distractions often occur during patient handoffs (Müller et al., 2018). For example, important information may not be included due to interruptions and distractions during the handoff. Since errors are often associated with miscommunication, strategies are needed to reduce errors when communicating during patient handoffs. Using simple communication tools can improve the handoff process. A standardized handoff tool allows for structured handoffs and minimizes the chance of omitting information. When used properly, I-PASS is a tool that may improve the handoff quality between health care team members (AHRQ, 2023b).

TABLE 3.2   **I-PASS Handoff Tool**

Illness Severity	• stable, "watcher," unstable
Patient Summary	• summary statement • events leading up to admissions or care transition • hospital course or treatment plan • ongoing assessment • contingency plan
Action List	• to-do list • timelines and ownership

(Continued)

Situation Awareness and Contingency Planning	• knowing what's going on • planning for what might happen
Synthesis by Receiver	• summary of what receiver heard • questions asked • restatement of key actions/to-do items

Electronic Health Records

EHRs can lead to improved communication among intraprofessional and interprofessional health care team members and improved patient care. *Intraprofessional communication* is communication between members of the same profession, while *interprofessional communication* is communication between members of two or more professions. When the EHR is functioning and used properly, it helps reduce fragmentation in care delivery. The shared health care information is precise and results in fewer errors in data sharing and higher quality outcomes (Janett & Yeracaris, 2020; Kruse et al., 2018). In addition, when an EHR is used correctly, it can decrease health care costs. Other benefits of proper EHR usage include increased self-care, quality of care, and health and patient-centered outcomes (Tapuria et al., 2021). An example of improved patient care based on EHR use is when patients miss a visit with their provider, their chart can be flagged, resulting in automatic reminders sent to the patient to reschedule the visit. EHRs can remind patients of the need for vaccines and routine screenings.

Another communication benefit of the EHR is the potential for patient engagement with the EHR and the health care team. Patients that use the EHR can communicate with their providers outside an office visit. Some patients prefer sending a brief message or question for minor concerns rather than scheduling an office visit. The EHR also provides advanced methods of delivering medication with accuracy and efficiency. The shared medication list on the EHR assists with care coordination along the continuum of care, resulting in fewer medication errors and better patient adherence and medication management (Janett & Yeracaris, 2020).

EHRs can also group patients according to needs to support data management and surveillance and to improve preventative care (Janett & Yeracaris, 2020). In turn, this supports programs that improve health outcomes, reduce health disparities for patients, and improves productivity and efficiency for health care professionals. For example, the health care team can use the EHR to identify patients at risk of developing diabetes, then reach out to each patient to offer referrals to resources such as nutrition or exercise programs.

The EHR improves access to health data for clinicians and researchers to understand better the health needs of patients and the greater community. By monitoring data sets of large groups of patients through the EHR, they can identify health concerns and preventative care needs in real time (Kruse et al., 2018). For example, by analyzing patient demographics, vital signs, laboratory data, and emergency room encounters, researchers can study the severity and progression of diseases and health issues within a population (Casey et al., 2016).

Artificial Intelligence and Communication

Artificial intelligence (AI) in health care is a tool to improve efficiency, alleviate workload, and reduce human error. More recently it has been recognized as having the potential to become a full-fledged member of the workplace team (Fischer, 2023). AI is used in health care to analyze data and information from the EHR and other sources and then communicate its findings to the health care team. For example, AI can "digitally read" a mammogram or EKG or identify a patient at risk of sepsis based on data entered into the EHR. AI is also used in diagnostic support systems to assist providers in making patient diagnoses (see Scenario 1). Often this works well because the AI systems can process large amounts of data and identify a potential diagnosis with accurate results. AI is used to communicate with patients through chatbots; the AI system can exchange text messages with patients, identify patients with more complex needs, and notify an HCP that the patient needs more specialized attention or education.

SCENARIO 1

Erika is an NP working at a retail clinic in October. Mr. Shor, age 50, comes in with a complaint of a cough. Erika knows that the flu has been common this fall and, before seeing him, decides to order a rapid flu test. She also orders a rapid COVID test. Both tests come back negative. Erika begins asking Mr. Shor questions to gather more information. He does not currently have a fever and has not had one recently. He states that he has been coughing more at night and that it may have started about a week ago, but it might have started before that. He is not aware of any exposures to the flu, COVID, or a cold, but he has been out in public and spending time with friends, so he may have been exposed without knowing.

When listening to his chest, Erika does not hear any unusual sounds. She is about to treat Mr. Shor for an upper respiratory illness and send him on his way. The EHR, which includes an AI-generated protocol list, indicates that Erika should ask questions regarding GERD (gastroesophageal reflux disease). Upon asking those questions, Erika learns that this often happens at night after Mr. Shor has had a large meal, which may have included an alcoholic drink. In addition, once or twice he has coughed up blood. Erika then believes that Mr. Shor has GERD, and because he has coughed up blood, she recommends that he take an over-the-counter H2 blocker such as famotidine (Pepcid). Then she gives him the name and number of a gastroenterologist to contact for follow-up. Erika heard from the patient several weeks later thanking her for her care because when he saw the gastroenterologist, he learned that he had Barrett's esophagitis. The combination of Erika's care and the AI protocol helped to get Mr. Shor the care he needed.

Despite the promising technology and recent advances in AI, there are still concerns. AI technology is imperfect (see Scenario 2 for an example), and individuals are still learning to trust it. People may need more time and experience using AI to fully trust and integrate it into their teams and workplaces (Lloyd & Khuman, 2022). Some HCPs are concerned that AI will replace them and that it will provide substandard care. However, one study of health care workers' jobs indicated that AI could do 40% of their work, leaving more time for interacting with patients (Burchardt & Aschenbrenner, 2023). The role of AI in health care will continue to evolve and grow over time. Nurses and other HCPs are essential in identifying how to use this technology to best improve patient care and the health care work environment. Whether AI remains a tool or becomes a full member of the interprofessional team, it will continue to influence how interprofessional teams communicate and work together.

SCENARIO 2

An oncology nurse, Maggie, was documenting in the EHR. An alert in the EHR indicated that Mr. Patel was septic and that the hospital's sepsis protocol should be initiated, which included significant blood work and antibiotics. Maggie knew his white blood cell count was high because of leukemia and not sepsis. She checked, and he had no fever or other signs of sepsis. The hospital policy required her to contact the physician to request that they override the sepsis treatment protocol. She tried several times but was unable to reach the physician. Maggie knew she could be written up if she did not follow sepsis protocol, so she reluctantly did so. When the blood work came back, the results indicated that Mr. Smith was not septic. Maggie stopped the antibiotics that were part of the sepsis protocol as they were unnecessary.

Discussion Questions

1. Compare how AI was used in both scenarios. What worked well? What could have worked better?
2. How was AI used to communicate in each scenario? What other types of communication were used in the scenario?
3. For each scenario, what is the responsibility of the NP or nurse to make sure AI is being applied appropriately? What is the responsibility of the retail clinic and the hospital?
4. What benefits and challenges do you see for patients and HCPs as AI becomes more integrated into health care?

Communication With Patients

Patients are an essential member of the interprofessional team. Basic communication skills are the same when communicating with patients and colleagues; however, some additional tools and strategies are better suited to patient interactions. HCPs frequently communicate verbally but are not always effective in getting their message across to patients. Careful and consistent communication improves the transfer of information. For example, faster rates of speech are significantly associated with the receiver understanding fewer words. Improving communication by slowing speech, using more understandable words, and intentionally allowing more time for patients to speak and ask questions may be immediate ways to help improve patient health outcomes (Rainey et al., 2022).

The Teach Back Method (see Figure 3.3) used to improve communication and understanding between the patient and HCP. This method allows the HCP to confirm that the patient understands essential information, as it asks the patient to describe information back to the educator or "teach back" in their own words (Burnett, 2021). If a patient has difficulty teaching back the information, the provider can reteach the concept using different words.

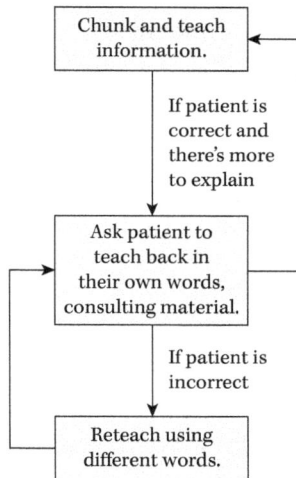

FIGURE 3.3   Teach-Back.

Barriers to Communication

To effectively communicate with patients and the health care team, HCPs need to understand factors that can pose barriers to communication. This section identifies some of the challenges to communication, and Table 3.3 outlines tips and resources to address those challenges.

PERSONAL PROTECTIVE EQUIPMENT

Personal protective equipment (PPE) undoubtedly protects health care professionals; however, PPE also presents difficulty with communication. Verbal communication is difficult, fatiguing, and frustrating while wearing PPE (Agarwal et al.,

2020; Schlögl et al., 2021). Face masks create a sound barrier and can soften a speaker's voice, conceal vocal tone, and hide facial expressions that relay essential nonverbal information. For many patients and caregivers, but specifically older adults, persons with cognitive impairment, and people who are hard of hearing, masks can limit communication, resulting in feelings of anxiety and stress. In addition, unfamiliar facial coverings can increase fear in children. A study that compared mask-wearing to nonmask-wearing physicians found that masks disrupt facial visual cues and significantly negatively impact perceptions of empathy (Wong et al., 2013).

CONFLICT

When conflict arises among health care team members, teamwork and communication can break down. Conflict can arise when team members have different opinions, ideas, or perceptions on completing a task or reaching a goal. A team can also experience interpersonal conflict, which arises between individuals on the team that is unrelated to the task at hand, but more to how the team members interact with each other (AHRQ, 2023c). In order to avoid communication breakdown among team members, it is crucial to identify and address the problem with timely feedback and conflict management (Epps & Levin, 2015). For more on conflict management, see Chapter 7.

HEALTH LITERACY

Healthy People 2030 identifies two types of health literacy: personal health literacy and organizational health literacy. Personal health literacy "is the degree to which individuals have the ability to find, understand, and use information and services to inform health-related decisions and actions for themselves and others" (Office of Disease Prevention and Health Promotion [ODPHP], n.d., para. 3). Personal health literacy strongly predicts health status

(Federico, 2014). People with limited health literacy can experience numerous adverse effects on their health. Someone with limited health literacy may not have the skills or knowledge to manage their care. For example, they may not understand the instructions provided for prescription medication. The patient may be unable to navigate the EHR or the health care system. These individuals are more likely to delay seeking health care, resulting in worse health outcomes than those with higher levels of health literacy (Levy & Janke, 2016).

Preventive care and services are often less utilized for someone with limited health literacy (Byrne, 2022). The individual may not know about the need and reason for preventative care, such as mammograms, colonoscopies, and annual physicals. They may also not know or understand when it is important to communicate with their HCP, which can put them at risk for more severe disease or hospital readmissions. When patients do not understand the reason for the health-related care or how to use the health information, they may engage less in their care and be less satisfied with the care they receive. HCPs need to assess their patient's health literacy level and health literacy practice universal precautions, meaning they assume all patients want easy-to-understand and comprehendible explanations (AHRQ, 2020b; Yim et al., 2018). When a patient is emotionally upset, no matter their health literacy level, they are at risk of misunderstanding health information.

Organizational health literacy "is the degree to which organizations equitably enable individuals to find, understand, and use information and services to inform health-related decisions and action for themselves and others" (ODPHP, n.d., para. 3). Health care organizations should work to address systemic barriers to health literacy such as the following:

- developing educational pamphlets, videos, and other materials so they are accessible to a wide range of reading levels

- training staff on how to assess individual health literacy and how to communicate effectively with people of different literacy levels
- ensuring that signs in the building and forms frequently used by patients are developed with health literacy in mind

In short, HCPs and health care organizations are responsible for creating systems that are easier for patients to understand and navigate. When assessing and working to improve organizational health literacy, patients and the rest of the interprofessional team are a good resource for understanding the organization's needs, barriers, and strengths related to health literacy (AHRQ, 2020a). Advanced nurses can play a role in this by leading efforts to improve organizational health literacy, evaluating health literacy programs, and advocating for local, state, or federal solutions to increase literacy rates.

LIMITED CULTURAL HUMILITY AND COMPETENCE

HCPs have a responsibility to learn how to work with their diverse patient population and their colleagues in a culturally sensitive way. Health care systems and professionals should be aware of and responsive to individuals' cultural perspectives and backgrounds, including language, cultural traditions, family preferences, values, and socioeconomic conditions (Stubbe, 2020). Being sensitive to cultural differences also includes understanding nonverbal language, such as eye contact, and lifestyle factors or personal circumstances that can influence and affect the plan of care. HCPs must also be aware of differences in professional cultures, values, beliefs, and attitudes (Bachynsky, 2019). For example, some health professional cultures may value a hierarchical structure for a team, while other professions emphasize more egalitarian team structures. The same skills apply to navigating cultural differences with patients or other HCPs.

Cultural competency and cultural humility are two common concepts discussed in health care. Cultural competency often refers to the idea that a person can gain the knowledge and skills to work effectively with people from different cultural backgrounds; it is often viewed as an endpoint. Cultural humility is often characterized more as an ongoing process rather than an endpoint. It includes self-reflection, openness, personal critique, partnering with patients and communities, and learning to understand better cultures outside of one's own (Stubbe, 2020; Tervalon & Murray-García, 1998). HCPs can incorporate both cultural competency and humility into their practice. HCPS must gain the knowledge and skills (competence) needed to work effectively with the people from the cultures they most often encounter in their work. Through cultural humility, they can build that competence, learn about more cultures, and avoid stereotyping patients or other HCPs (Stubbe, 2020). An important step in this process is understanding one's own implicit biases; for more on implicit bias see Chapter 6.

LANGUAGE BARRIERS

With increased global migration, language barriers in health care have become more prevalent. The language barrier can affect many aspects of patient care, including but not limited to health care access, patient satisfaction, health outcomes, cost, and safety (Squires, 2018). Medical interpreters can help connect patients and clinicians. In 1964, the U.S. Civil Rights Act helped to ensure that limited English proficient (LEP) persons would have legal protections against discrimination. Title VI of the Civil Rights Act of 1964 prohibited discrimination against LEP persons based on national origin. Health and social service providers are required to take adequate steps to ensure that such persons receive the language assistance necessary to afford them meaningful access to their services free of charge (U.S. Department of Health and

Human Services, 2000). Unfortunately, HCPs do not consistently use interpreting services when patients need them (O'Toole et al., 2019). Integrating an interpreter into regular care can be challenging and takes planning on the part of the HCP and the health care institution. When used effectively and consistently, interpreting services improves patient care and satisfaction.

Professional interpreters in health care settings typically have been trained in interpreting medical information and may have additional cultural knowledge they can share with the health care team (Squires, 2018). For example, a medical interpreter ensures that health information is delivered using culturally specific phrasing that the patient may better understand. Interpreters can work on-site, in person, over the telephone, or by video conferencing. Interpreting refers to spoken language, while translating refers to converting written information from one language to another. Interpreting and translating require different skills, so it is important for health care organizations and HCPs not to rely on interpreters to translate documents, particularly if they have not had the time to review the document ahead of time and if the document is lengthy (O'Toole et al., 2019). For tips on how to work with interpreters and LEP see Table 3.3.

TABLE 3.3   **Tips and Resources to Address Communication Barriers**

Communication Barrier	Tips and Resources
PPE	• Wear large written name tag. • Use a higher tone of voice. • Speak slowly. • User clear and concise terminology. • Repeat concepts several times. • Ask for teach-back or closed-loop. • Use a calm voice during procedures (Ferrari et al., 2021).

Communication Barrier	Tips and Resources
Conflict	• Identify and address the problem with timely feedback and conflict resolution. • Ensure all team members have the necessary information to complete their assigned role. • Team members can ask for and offer assistance so that the team can work together instead of against one another (Epps & Levin, 2015).
Individual health literacy	• Assess the patient's health literacy level. • Speak slowly and carefully. • Use teach-back and show-back. • Ask open-ended questions. • Use graphics instead of lengthy written explanations (Federico, 2014). University of Maryland, Health Literacy Resources: https://guides.hshsl.umaryland.edu/healthliteracy/assessment This website provides a list of resources and tools to assess individual health literacy and readability of health education materials.
Organizational health literacy	AHRQ Health Literacy Universal Precautions Toolkit (2nd ed.): https://www.ahrq.gov/health-literacy/improve/precautions/index.html CDC Health Literacy: https://www.cdc.gov/healthliteracy/researchevaluate/index.html Healthy People 2030: Evidence-Based Resources: https://health.gov/healthypeople/tools-action/browse-evidence-based-resources U.S Department of Health and Human Services, National Action Plan to Improve Health Literacy: https://health.gov/our-work/national-health-initiatives/health-literacy/national-action-plan-improve-health-literacy

(Continued)

Communication Barrier	Tips and Resources
Limited cultural humility and competence	For individual HCPs: • Ask the individual about their identity and personal a lives. Don't assume. • Listen more than you speak. • Engage in self-reflection on your own identity and beliefs. • Recognize that disease may not be the only issue for the patient. • Learn about the cultures with which you frequently come into contact. • Learn about the communities where your patients live. • Approach patients and colleagues with an open mind, genuine curiosity, and interest (McGee-Avila, 2018; Stubbe, 2020). For health care organizations: • Collect relevant demographic data such as race, ethnicity, and language preference. • Identify and report disparities. • Create culturally competent programs. • Provide culturally and linguistically competent care. • Engage the community. • Work to increase the diversity of your workforce. • Prioritize cultural competency in your organization (American Hospital Association, n.d.).
Language barriers	• Offer language assistance for individuals with language or other communication needs. • Inform all individuals of language assistance options. • Use competent individuals for language assistance, avoiding untrained individuals or minors. • Provide print materials and signage in the languages commonly used by the populations in the service area. • Provide sensitivity to cultural differences during patient interactions (U.S. Department of Health & Human Services, 2022).

Communication Barrier	Tips and Resources
Working with interpreters	• Include the interpreter as part of the care team; when possible, talk with them before and after the patient encounter to brief and debrief the situation. • If in person, look at and talk directly to the patient as you would if the interpreter was not there. Avoid talking only to the interpreter when the message is intended for the patient. • If on a phone or video call, limit background noise, speak clearly, and pause frequently to allow time for questions. • Only talk about the information you want to discuss with the patient while working with an interpreter. Avoid side conversations; the interpreter must translate everything spoken while the patient is present. • If you do not feel confident the interpreter is conveying the information accurately, pause and confirm the content of the message with them. Use the time with the interpreter effectively; allow time for the patient to ask questions or communicate other needs while the interpreter is available (O'Toole et al., 2019; Squires, 2018).

SCENARIO 3

Mr. Brosz, an 84-year-old widower, was brought to the emergency department (ED) by the local emergency medical services (EMS). Mr. Brosz lives alone in a senior high-rise. He has three children. His daughter Nancy and her family live nearby. His son, Thomas, also lives within 30 minutes of his father, and his youngest daughter, Janet, lives in another state and has a 12-hour drive to her father's home. Janet and her family usually visit for the holidays.

Mr. Brosz called the EMS because he had increased shortness of breath, dizziness, and a change in mental status. When Mr. Brosz arrived in the ED he was unresponsive, his breathing was labored, and he had a strong pulse.

The apartment management notified Thomas that his father was taken to the local hospital. Thomas arrived at the hospital shortly after Mr. Brosz arrived at the ED. The medical team began to ask Thomas if his father has a medical power of attorney or living will. Thomas said he was unsure, but he knew his sister, Janet, took care of the "legal stuff." Thomas also said his father would want "everything done to keep him alive." The case manager arrived and reviewed documentation in the EHR from a prior hospitalization. She found a document indicating that Mr. Brosz requested a do not attempt to resuscitate (DNAR) order, which was placed during his last hospitalization. The case manager asked Thomas about the prior DNAR order. Thomas was surprised and emphasized that his dad was only 84 years old and would want to be there for his children and grandchildren. He was certain his dad would want everything done to remain alive. The case manager contacted Janet. Janet indicated that she had medical power of attorney papers, and her father did request the DNAR order. She would fax the paperwork to the hospital after she finished work. Janet was certain that her dad did not want to be on life support. Mr. Brosz was admitted to the ICU for further care.

Mr. Brosz was rapidly declining, and a treatment decision was needed. The medical team began to discuss the goals of care and possible treatment options. At this time, no legal documents were available to the medical team identifying a medical power of attorney. Nancy and Thomas were present in the ICU, and they agreed that their dad would want everything done to sustain life. The medical team decided to intubate Mr. Brosz. After the procedure was complete, the unit clerk came to the room and stated that Janet was on the phone and wanted to talk with a team member regarding her father's care. The NP took the phone call and shared with Janet that her father was in critical condition and the reasons there was a need for life-sustaining treatment. Janet emphatically stated she was the medical power of attorney and her father had conversations with her, indicating that he did not want life-sustaining measures for religious reasons. Janet stated that her father was concerned that Nancy and Thomas might disagree with his choices, especially her father's rationale related to his religion.

Janet faxed a copy of the medical power of attorney to the hospital. When the document was received, the medical team agreed that the documents were legitimate and that Janet was the contact person for further care related to Mr. Brosz. Janet requested that the medical team and family have a phone or video meeting to discuss her father's status and plan of care. The NP and pastoral care provider agreed to meet with the family. The attending physician from the ICU was not available to meet. At the request of the NP, the palliative medicine physician agreed to also be present during the family meeting. The team meeting results in the decision to extubate Mr. Brosz and provide symptom management and end-of-life care. Mr. Brosz died within hours of Janet and her family arriving at the hospital. The family received bereavement support through the hospital. The ICU nurse manager suggested that the team members conduct a formal debriefing to discuss the care of Mr. Brosz.

Discussion Questions

1. Identify all the people involved in communicating in this scenario.
2. What forms of communication do they use?
3. What were some of the barriers to communication?
4. What was done well, and what could be done to improve communication in this situation?

CONCLUSION

The strategies to facilitate communication and the barriers identified in this chapter are a few examples of the complexity that nurses, patients, and other HCPs face when trying to communicate with each other. Effective communication is an ongoing process, a skill that can be learned and improved upon over time. Nurses can lead by example by practicing effective communication skills with patients and their team members using strategies such as huddles, briefs, debriefs, closed-loop communication, and standardized handoffs. They can lead their organizations to make system-level improvements to facilitate good communication with patients and among team members, through EHRs, AI, and other technologies, as well as developing policies and procedures that support clear communication among team members. Good communication is central to quality patient care, and all members of the interprofessional team hold the responsibility to develop the skills needed to communicate effectively with each other.

KEY POINTS

- Effective communication between interprofessional team members and patients is essential to providing safe care.
- Structured communication tools can help improve health care team communication to reduce medical errors, conflict, and misunderstandings.
- Existing and emerging technologies, such as the EHR and AI, play an important role in how HCPs communicate with each other and with patients.
- To communicate effectively, nurses must understand the communication barriers and how to prevent or address them if they arise.

ACTIVITIES

Activity 1: Brief and Debrief Checklists

Imagine that you are called on to lead a brief and debrief for the situation described in Scenario 3. Use the Brief and Debrief Checklist in the TeamSTEPPS Pocket Guide found here: https://www.ahrq.gov/teamstepps-program/resources/pocket-guide/index.html. For the brief, imagine you are on the ICU team and have to brief your team about Mr. Jackson after he was transferred from the ED before he was intubated. Answer the questions on the brief checklist as best as you can. Now imagine you are leading the debrief for the team after Mr. Jackson's death. Review and answer the questions on the debrief checklist as best you can.

DISCUSSION QUESTIONS

1. What checklist items were easy to answer?

2. What other information did you need to complete the checklist? Where might you find that type of information in a real-life situation?

3. When would it be an appropriate time for the team to call a huddle during this scenario? Who should call the huddle in that situation?

Activity 2: Interactive Teach-Back Learning Module

Complete the Interactive Teach-back Learning Module available here: http://www.teachbacktraining.org/interactive-teach-back-learning-module.

The module takes about 45 minutes to complete and has two parts:

- It describes teach-back and demonstrates its effectiveness as a health literacy intervention to improve patient–provider communication.
- Video and interactive self-assessment questions enhance, confirm, and reinforce your ability to use teach-back and integrate it into your clinical practice.

Activity 3: Reflection: Professional Cultures, Cultural Humility, and Cultural Competence

Take time to reflect on how you perceive the professional culture of nursing. What are the values, beliefs, and ideas that many nurses hold in common? Identify a person who is working in a non-nursing profession. This person could be a friend, coworker, family member, or staff member at your clinical site. They do not have to be a health professional. Interview this person about their perspective on their profession's culture, using the tips for improving cultural humility and competence listed in Table 3.3.

DISCUSSION QUESTIONS

1. What did you learn about this person's professional culture?

2. What are the similarities and differences between this person's professional culture and your perception of nursing's professional culture?

3. How was this similar or different from learning about a patient's culture?

REFERENCES

Agarwal, A., Agarwal, S., & Motiani, P. (2020). Difficulties encountered while using PPE kits and how to overcome them: An Indian perspective. *Cureus*, *12*(11), e11652. https://doi.org/10.7759/cureus.11652

Agency for Healthcare Research and Quality. (2020a). *Form a team: Tool #1. Health Literacy Universal Precautions Toolkit* (2nd ed.). https://www.ahrq.gov/health-literacy/improve/precautions/tool1.html

Agency for Healthcare Research and Quality. (2020b). *AHRQ health literacy universal precautions toolkit*. https://www.ahrq.gov/health-literacy/improve/precautions/index.html

Agency for Healthcare Research and Quality. (2023a). *Module 2: Team leadership, section 1: Overview of key concepts and tools*. https://www.ahrq.gov/teamstepps-program/curriculum/team/overview/index.html

Agency for Healthcare Research and Quality. (2023b). *Module 1: Communication, section 1: Overview of key concepts and tools*. https://www.ahrq.gov/teamstepps-program/curriculum/communication/overview/index.html

Agency for Healthcare Research and Quality. (2023c). *Module 4: Mutual support, concept: Conflict in teams*. https://www.ahrq.gov/teamstepps-program/curriculum/mutual/tools/conflict.html

American Association of Colleges of Nursing. (2021). *The essentials: Core competencies for professional nursing education*. https://www.aacnnursing.org/AACN-Essentials/Download

American Hospital Association. (n.d.). *Becoming a culturally competent healthcare organization*. https://www.aha.org/ahahret-guides/2013-06-18-becoming-culturally-competent-health-care-organization

Bachynsky, N. (2019). Implications for policy: The triple aim, quadruple aim, and interprofessional collaboration. *Nursing Forum*, *55*(1), 54–64. https://doi.org/10.1111/nuf.12382

Boss, R. D., Hirschfeld, R. S., Barone, S., Johnson, E., & Arnold, R. M. (2020). Pediatric chronic critical illness: Training teams to address the communication challenges of patients with repeated and prolonged hospitalizations. *Journal of Pain and Symptom Management, 60*(5), 959–967. https://doi.org/10.1016/j.jpainsymman.2020.06.005

Burchardt, A., & Aschenbrenner, D. (2023). Practical guide AI=all together and interdisciplinary. In I. Knappertsbusch & K. Gondlach (Eds.), *Work and AI: Challenges and strategies for tomorrow's work* (pp. 11–19). Springer. https://doi.org/10.1007/978-3-658-40232-7

Burnett, B. (2021, September 3). *Understanding the teach-back method.* STAR Center. https://star-center.org/understanding-the-teach-back-method/

Byrne D. (2022). Understanding and mitigating low health literacy. *Nursing Standard (Royal College of Nursing), 37*(10), 27–34. https://doi.org/10.7748/ns.2022.e11875

Casey, J. A., Schwartz, B. S., Stewart, W. F., & Adler, N. E. (2016). Using electronic health records for population health research: a review of methods and applications. *Annual Review of Public Health, 31*(1). 61–81. https://doi.org/10.1146/annurev-publhealth-032315-021353

Crowe, C. A. (2017). Communication. In P. A. Potter, A. G. Perry, P. A. Stockert, & A. M. Hall (Eds.), *Fundamentals of nursing* (9th ed., pp. 316–335). Elsevier.

Dahlke, S., Hunter, K., Reshef Kalogirou, M., Negrin, K., Fox, M., & Wagg, A. (2020). Perspectives about interprofessional collaboration and patient-centred care. *Canadian Journal on Aging / La Revue Canadienne Du Vieillissement, 39*(3), 443–455. https://doi.org/10.1017/S0714980819000539

Epps, H. R., & Levin, P. E. (2015). The TeamSTEPPS approach to safety and quality. *Journal of Pediatric Orthopaedics, 35*, S30–S33. https://doi.org/10.1097/bpo.0000000000000541

Federico, F. (2014). *8 ways to improve health literacy.* Institute for Healthcare Improvement. https://www.ihi.org/communities/blogs/8-ways-to-improve-health-literacy#:~:text=Speak%20more%20slowly%20when%20providing

Ferrari, G., Dobrina, R., Buchini, S., Rudan, I., Schreiber, S., & Bicego, L. (2021). The impact of personal protective equipment and social distancing on communication and relation between nurses, caregivers and children: A descriptive qualitative study in a maternal and child health hospital. *Journal of Clinical Nursing.* https://doi.org/10.1111/jocn.15857

Fischer, F. (2023). Future collaboration between humans and AI. In I. Knappertsbusch & K. Gondlach (Eds.), *Work and AI: Challenges and strategies for tomorrow's work* (pp. 21–28) Springer. https://doi.org/10.1007/978-3-658-40232-7

Janett, R., & Yeracaris, P. (2020). Electronic medical records in the American health system: Challenges and lessons learned. *Ciencia*

& *Saude Coletiva*, *25*(4), 1293–1304. https://doi.org/10.1590/1413-81232020254.28922019

Kruse, C. S., Stein, A., Thomas, H., & Kaur, H. (2018). The use of electronic health records to support population health: A systematic review of the literature. *Journal of Medical Systems*, *42*(11), 214. https://doi.org/10.1007/s10916-018-1075-6

Levy, H., & Janke, A. (2016). Health literacy and access to care. *Journal of Health Communication*, *21*(1), 43–50. https://doi.org/10.1080/10810730.2015.1131776

Lloyd, N., & Khuman, A.S. (2022). *AI in healthcare: Malignant or benign?* In T. Chen, J. Carter, M. Mahmud, & A. S. Khuman (Eds.), *Artificial intelligence in health care: Recent applications and developments* (pp. 1–45). Springer. https://doi.org/10.1007/978-981-19-5272-2

McGee-Avila, J. (2018, June 21). *Practicing cultural humility to transform health care.* Robert Wood Johnson Foundation. https://www.rwjf.org/en/insights/blog/2018/06/practicing-cultural-humility-to-transform-health-care.html#:~:text=Listen%20More%20Than%20You%20Speak,to%20achieve%20their%20health%20goals

Müller, M., Jürgens, J., Redaèlli, M., Klingberg, K., Hautz, W. E., & Stock, S. (2018). Impact of the communication and patient hand-off tool SBAR on patient safety: a systematic review. *BMJ Open*, *8*(8), e022202. https://doi.org/10.1136/bmjopen-2018-022202

Newell, S., & Jordan, Z. (2015). The patient experience of patient-centered communication with nurses in the hospital setting: A qualitative systematic review protocol. *JBI Database of Systematic reviews and Implementation Reports*, *13*(1), 76–87.https://doi.org/10.11124/jbisrir-2015-1072

Office of Disease Prevention and Health Promotion. (n.d.). Health literacy in Healthy People 2023. *Healthy People 2030.* U.S. Department of Health and Human Services. https://health.gov/healthypeople/priority-areas/health-literacy-healthy-people-2030

O'Toole, J. K., Alvarado-Little, W., & Ledford, C. J. W. (2019). Communication with diverse patients: Addressing culture and language. *Pediatric Clinics of North America*, *66*(4), 791–804. https://doi.org/10.1016/j.pcl.2019.03.006

Parker, A. L., Forsythe, L. L., & Kohlmorgen, I. K. (2019). TeamSTEPPS®: An evidence-based approach to reduce clinical errors threatening safety in outpatient settings: An integrative review. *Journal of Healthcare Risk Management: The Journal of the American Society for Healthcare Risk Management*, *38*(4), 19–31. https://doi.org/10.1002/jhrm.21352

Purnell, L. (2018). Cross cultural communication: Verbal and non-verbal communication, interpretation and translation. In M. M. Douglas, D. Pacquiao, & L. Purnell (Eds.), *Global applications of culturally competent health care: Guidelines for practice* (pp. 131–142). Springer. https://doi.org/10.1007/978-3-319-69332-3_14

Rainey, R., Theiss, L., Lopez, E., Wood, T., Wood, L., Marques, I., Cannon, J. A., Kennedy, G. D., Morris, M. S., Hollis, R., Davis, T., & Chu, D. I. (2022). Characterizing the impact of verbal communication and health literacy in the patient-surgeon encounter. *American Journal of Surgery*, *224*(3), 943–948. https://doi.org/10.1016/j.amjsurg.2022.04.034

Schlögl, M., Singler, K., Martinez-Velilla, N., Jan, S., Bischoff-Ferrari, H. A., Roller-Wirnsberger, R. E., Attier-Zmudka, J., Jones, C. A., Miot, S., & Gordon, A. L. (2021). Communication during the COVID-19 pandemic: Evaluation study on self-perceived competences and views of health care professionals. *European Geriatric Medicine*, *12*(6), 1181–1190. https://doi.org/10.1007/s41999-021-00532-1

Sibiya, M. N. (2018). Effective communication in nursing. *InTech*. https://doi.org/10.5772/intechopen.74995

Squires A. (2018). Strategies for overcoming language barriers in healthcare. *Nursing Management*, *49*(4), 20–27. https://doi.org/10.1097/01.NUMA.00005311

Stubbe, D. E. (2020). Practicing cultural competence and cultural humility in the care of diverse patients. *Focus*, *18*(1), 49–51. https://doi.org/10.1176/appi.focus.20190041

Tapuria, A., Porat, T., Kalra, D., Dsouza, G., Xiaohui, S., & Curcin, V. (2021). Impact of patient access to their electronic health record: Systematic review. *Informatics for Health & Social Care*, *46*(2), 192–204. https://doi.org/10.1080/17538157.2021.1879810

Tervalon, M., & Murray-García, J. (1998). Cultural humility versus cultural competence: A critical distinction in defining physician training outcomes in multicultural education. *Journal of Health Care for the Poor and Underserved*, *9*(2), 117–125. https://doi.org/10.1353/hpu.2010.0233

Thakur, K., & Sharma, S. K. (2021). Nurse with smile: Does it make difference in patients' healing? *Industrial Psychiatry Journal*, *30*(1), 6–10. https://doi.org/10.4103/ipj.ipj_165_20

University of Maryland Health Sciences and Human Services Library. (2023). *Health literacy resources: Assessment.* https://guides.hshsl.umaryland.edu/healthliteracy/assessment

U.S. Department of Health and Human Services (2000). Title VI of Civil Right Act of 1964; policy guidance on the prohibition against national origin discrimination as it affects persons with limited English proficiency. *Federal Register*, *65*(169). 52762-52774. https://www.federalregister.gov/documents/2000/08/30/00-22140/title-vi-of-the-civil-rights-act-of-1964-policy-guidance-on-the-prohibition-against-national-origin

van Manen, A. S., Aarts, S., Metzelthin, S. F., Verbeek, H., Hamers, J. P. H., & Zwakhalen, S. M. G. (2021). A communication model for nursing staff working in dementia care: Results of a scoping review. *International Journal of Nursing Studies*, *113*, 103776. https://doi.org/10.1016/j.ijnurstu.2020.103776

Werder O. (2019). Toward a humanistic model in health communication. *Global Health Promotion, 26*(1), 33–40. https://doi.org/10.1177/1757975916683385

Wong, C. K., Yip, B. H., Mercer, S., Griffiths, S., Kung, K., Wong, M. C., Chor, J., & Wong, S. Y. (2013). Effect of facemasks on empathy and relational continuity: a randomized controlled trial in primary care. *BMC Family Practice, 14*, 200. https://doi.org/10.1186/1471-2296-14-200

Yim, C. K., Shumate, L., Barnett, S. H., & Leitman, I. M. (2018). Health literacy assessment and patient satisfaction in surgical practice. *Annals of Medicine and Surgery, 35*, 25–28. https://doi.org/10.1016/j.amsu.2018.08.022

CREDITS

CHAPTER 4

Effective Role Performance

Kristina Banks, DNP, APRN, CPNP-PC, and Mary de Haan, MSN, RN, ACNS-BC, CNE

KEY AACN COMPETENCIES, SUB-COMPETENCIES, AND CONCEPTS

Domain 2: Person-Centered Care

Competency 2.5 Develop a plan of care.

- **Advanced-Level Sub-Competency 2.5h** Lead and collaborate with an interprofessional team to develop a comprehensive plan of care.

Domain 5: Quality and Safety

Competency 5.3 Contribute to a culture of provider and work environment safety.

- **Entry-Level Sub-Competency 5.3d** Recognize one's role in sustaining a just culture reflecting civility and respect.

Domain 6: Interprofessional Partnerships

Competency 6.2 Perform effectively in different team roles, using principles and values of team dynamics.

- **Entry-Level Sub-Competency 6.2d** Recognize how one's uniqueness (as a person and a nurse) contributes to effective interprofessional working relationships.
- **Advanced-Level Sub-Competency 6.2i** Reflect on how one's role and expertise influences team performance.

Continued

Continued

> **Domain 10: Personal, Professional, and Leadership Development**
>
> • **Competency 10.2** Demonstrate a spirit of inquiry that fosters flexibility and professional maturity.
> • **Entry-Level Sub-Competency 10.2b** Integrate comprehensive feedback to improve performance.

KEY TERMS

Team	Team dynamics
Interprofessional team	Organizational culture
Interprofessional teamwork	Just culture
Spirit of inquiry	Comprehensive plan of care
Expertise	Imposter syndrome
Collaboration	

INTRODUCTION: EFFECTIVE PERFORMANCE OF ROLE

Interprofessional teams are a powerful strategy to address the increasingly complex health care environment in the United States and globally (Institute of Medicine, 2015). Though the United States spends more per capita on health care, its citizens consistently have worse health outcomes than other industrialized nations (Dingel et al. n.d.; National Academies of Sciences, Engineering, and Medicine, 2011). Health care inequities continue to negatively impact the health of individuals, families, and communities. Health care systems and providers must work together as a team in order to address factors ranging from health policy, technology, and social determinants of health that impact the individuals and communities they serve in order to deliver safe, equitable, quality care (National Academies of Sciences, Engineering, and Medicine, 2021). Nurses representing the majority of health care providers in the workforce, are "uniquely positioned to manage teams and link clinical care, public health, and social services" (National Academies of Sciences, Engineering, and Medicine, 2011, p. 4) and play a critical role on interprofessional teams (Balmer, 2020). The tenets of nursing practice, described in the American Nurses Association's (ANA, 2015) Scope and Standards of Practice, highlight the ability of nurses to establish partnerships with both consumers and providers of health care when planning and providing safe, quality care. The key concepts and competencies associated with a nurse's effective performance of role on an interprofessional team will be described here.

One example of how health care teams can improve patient care is by collaborating on a comprehensive plan of care. A comprehensive plan of care is a "dynamic [document] maintained by an interdisciplinary team that [contains] specific, actionable information for clinicians and staff across multiple care settings" (Theodorou et al., 2020). Patients with complex and diverse needs, in particular, require such a comprehensive plan. All nurses are active collaborators on the comprehensive plan of care. Additionally, according to the American Association of Colleges of Nursing (AACN) competency 2.5h, an APRN should both "lead and collaborate with an interprofessional team to develop a comprehensive plan of care" (AACN, 2021).

To be effective, interprofessional teams must have the ability to optimize and monitor the performance of their team members, which includes having a clear understanding of individual scopes of practice, levels of expertise, and unique individual contributions to the team (Krivanek et al., 2020; von der Lancken & Gunn, 2018). *Team dynamics* describe how a team interacts, communicates, works together, and influences the efficacy of the team (Belker et al., 2019). Mutual trust, adaptability, clear and transparent communication, and shared goals reflect a high degree of team effectiveness (Birnback & Salas, 2020; Frankel et al., 2017). Teams that communicate effectively and have mutual support reduce potential errors, improve clinical performance, and enhance patient safety (Health Research & Educational Trust, 2015).

When an interprofessional team is indicated, what is the role of the nurse on the team? *Team roles* are the responsibilities assigned to or associated with a person's position on a team. One approach to team roles is based on individual competencies. From this perspective, there is a defined set of attributes, knowledge, or skills of each health care provider required for collaborative practice (McLaney et al., 2022). The nurse's role on an interprofessional team, from this perspective, may be delineated by the ANA. The definition of nursing according to the ANA (2015) is "the protection, promotion, and optimization of health and abilities; prevention of illness and injury; facilitation of healing; alleviation of suffering through the diagnosis and treatment of human response; and advocacy in the care of individuals, families, groups, communities, and populations" (p. 7). This definition, encompassing both the role of the registered nurse (RN) and the advanced practice registered nurse (APRN), requires nurses to be well versed in communication, collaboration, care planning and delivery, and resource utilization (ANA, 2015). Nurses are clinicians, educators, advocates, researchers, and change agents—all roles motivated by a *spirit of inquiry*. This characteristic can be described as "a consistent, intentional, and applied professional curiosity" (Harper et al., 2019, p. 49) and "an ongoing curiosity about the best evidence to guide clinical decision making" (Melnyk et al., 2009, p. 119). One may describe a spirit of inquiry as being cognitively flexible and motivated by gaining new insight more than by defending one's own position. This encourages nurses to "explore, investigate, and assess" their roles and responsibilities within the interprofessional health care team, with the intention of promoting evidence-based care practices" (Koehne, 2018). The team role approach based on individual competencies has been used as a framework for standards of practice, to support the knowledge and skills of health care professionals, or to set performance indicators used for evaluation of ability to practice collaboratively (McLaney et al., 2022). Within this perspective, the assumption is that if each individual meets their competencies, the interprofessional collaboration and team performance will be optimal (McLaney et al., 2022). However, this brings us back to the distinction between a multidisciplinary rather than interprofessional team approach. An effective interprofessional team's success is based on the collective efforts of team members, through shared responsibility and collaborative decision-making (McLaney et al., 2022). To this end, team-based competencies for interprofessional collaboration may be considered. One such example is the Sunnybrook competency framework, developed by an interprofessional working group at Sunnybrook Health Sciences Centre, an academic medical center in Toronto, Ontario, and the largest trauma center in Canada. The Sunnybrook competency framework promotes collective competence rather than individual capabilities and will be described in more detail in the Team Roles, Team Dynamics, and Team Performance section of this chapter.

Another perspective for team roles is based on expertise, defined as expert knowledge or skill in a particular subject, activity, or job (Oxford Advanced Learner's Dictionary, 2023). Specific to nursing expertise, the foundation for development of the nursing role begins in nursing education and progresses with the development of experience and expertise in practice. It is important to note that expertise is based on many different aspects and is therefore fluid, variable, and situation specific. One may have professional knowledge that lends them expertise in specific scenarios but novice status in different environments. On an interprofessional team, the person with the least academic expertise may be the most expert at interpersonal communication. For example, a newly graduated RN may have come from a large family, and she became expert at navigating the demands of multiple perspectives, opinions, and personalities. She may therefore be better equipped than a more veteran member of the team at communicating the comprehensive care plan to the patient and their family. As a member of an interprofessional team, it is important for each individual to assess their own expertise in order to improve *team dynamics* and *team performance*. Team dynamics are the behavioral relationships between members of a given team. Team performance is how successful a team is, or how well they do what they set out to do (Collins Dictionary, 2023). According to Zajac et al. (2021), team performance reflects "individual and team-level teamwork, task-work, and team level processes that arise when working toward a shared goal" (p. 3) Health Research & Educational Trust (2015) notes that teams that communicate effectively and have mutual support reduce potential errors, enhance patient safety, and improve clinical performance.

Quality and safety is AACN's Domain 5. Competency 5.3 is to "contribute to a culture of provider and work environment safety." One way this is done is to "recognize one's role in sustaining a just culture reflecting civility and respect" (5.3d). *Just culture* utilizes "non-blaming error reporting systems to improve safety and reliability" (Paradiso & Sweeney, 2019) and "strives to make care as safe as it can be" (Health Quality Council of Alberta, 2023). Components of a just culture include building trust by treating individuals within the organization with respect and dignity while holding people accountable for their actions without making rash judgments (Health Quality Council of Alberta, 2023). Just culture is a subset of *organizational culture*, which includes the shared attitudes, values, and practices of an organization that frames the approach interprofessional teams use when interacting with each other, when learning from experiences, and when engaging with stakeholders, patients, and families (Frankel et al., 2017).

APPLICATIONS

Just Culture and Safety

Consider the various health care settings in which interprofessional teams function. Each has its own unique composition and organizational culture. Historically, the role of the nurse in maintaining a safe environment for patients has been viewed as foundational to the practice of nursing. Nurses were seen as solely responsible for maintaining infection control principles, accurately administering medications, and assuring that the overall patient environment was free from hazards. Armstrong (2019) asserts that this mind-set is changing to frame nursing practice as a "more complex, multifaceted phenomenon" (p. 444). Patient assessment, situation monitoring, clear and timely communication, and evaluation of outcomes are interwoven into what it means to "maintain a safe environment." Delivering quality care and maintaining patient safety are not unique to the role of nurses, but rather are the shared responsibility of the interprofessional team. The just culture framework places emphasis on how to improve the system of care delivery rather than on errors or negative outcomes (Armstrong, 2019). Understanding not only design flaws within the organization that lead to error, but the behavioral choices made by persons can lead to meaningful improvements to improve patient safety (Paradiso & Sweeney, 2019). Understanding whether an error occurred due to an inadvertent mistake versus situations in which the person is either unaware or intentionally disregards the potential risks of

Sub-Competency 5.3d: Recognize One's Role in Sustaining a Just Culture Reflecting Civility and Respect

SCENARIO 1

David is an experienced RN working on a general medical surgical unit that has been chronically short staffed. The morning is starting out very chaotic, with new admissions coming to the unit while other patients are leaving for surgery. In between receiving shift report and answering the unit phone, David needs to administer morning insulin doses to three separate patients by 0700 prior to breakfast service. The hospital has a policy in place for administration of high-risk medications, requiring two RNs to verify insulin dosages before administration. David, feeling confident in his skills and feeling rushed, draws up the insulin dose for the first patient without verification from a second nurse and administers the dose. When he returns to the medication cart to prepare the next dose, he realizes he was looking at the wrong medication record and inadvertently gave the patient the insulin dose intended for the third patient in his assignment. David notifies the patient's attending physician and his nurse manager, who instructs him to complete an incident report before meeting to debrief the situation. David is angry at himself for potentially causing harm to his patient and for not following hospital protocol, but even more so at the circumstances that led to his actions.

Discussion Questions

1. A just culture mind-set aims to examine the circumstances that lead to negative outcomes as one step toward improving care delivery. Identify the systemic and individual factors in this scenario that contributed to this medication error.
2. Compare and contrast how the debriefing meeting would proceed in an organization that has implemented a just culture approach versus one without.
3. Medical errors can have a devastating effect on a nurse's self-confidence. How can David's nurse manager support him at this time?
4. How should the medication error be addressed with the patient?

a situation helps frame the approach to corrective actions (Paradiso & Sweeney, 2019). With these factors in mind, organizations need to create and support a psychologically safe environment in which questions, suggestions, and ideas for improvement are welcomed and medical errors or near-miss events are viewed as opportunities for learning and system evaluation (Frankel et al., 2017). Without a sense of psychological safety, team members are less likely to speak up, to ask questions, or to make suggestions for improvement (O'Donovan & McAuliffe, 2020). Positive relationships, connectivity, and respect shared by team members builds confidence and promotes interprofessional collaboration, which ultimately positively impacts patient safety and health outcomes (Furr et al., 2020). For more on psychological safety see Chapter 7.

Team Roles, Team Dynamics, and Team Performance

The concept of teamwork in health care was refined in a 2005 collaboration between the Agency for Healthcare Research and Quality and the U.S. Department of Defense coined TeamSTEPPS©—Team Strategies and Tools to Enhance Performance and Patient Safety. TeamSTEPPS© includes a safety tool kit that "helps organizations improve the quality, safety and efficiency of health care delivery" (Health Research & Educational Trust, 2015, p. 4, pp2). Principle-based team training programs, such as TeamSTEPPS©, have been found to enhance interprofessional team skills, specifically team behavior, communication, and clarity of roles and responsibilities (Buljac-Samardzic et al., 2020).

The TeamSTEPPS© framework (Figure 4.1) is based on four core competencies: communication, leadership, situation monitoring, and mutual support (Health Research & Educational Trust, 2015). The TeamSTEPPS© competencies help to describe AACN's Competency 6.2, "principles and values of team dynamics." According to TeamSTEPPS©, communication is the effective exchange of information among team members. Leadership includes direction and

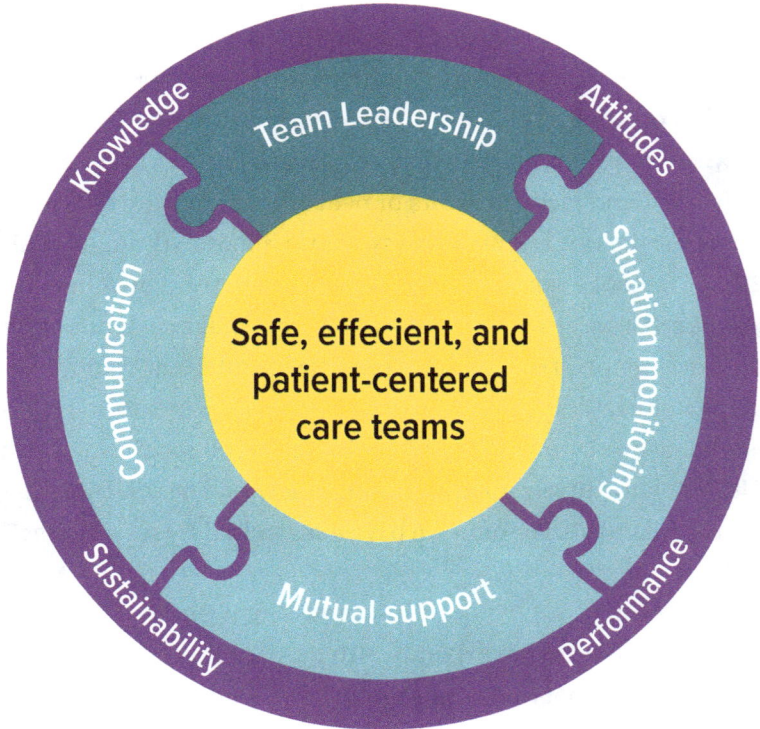

FIGURE 4.1 TeamSTEPPS® logo.

coordination, the assigning of tasks, motivating team members, and facilitating optimal performance. Situation monitoring is the development of common understandings of team environment, applying strategies for monitoring team members' performance, and maintaining a "shared mental model." A shared mental model involves all members of the team maintaining awareness of the situation at hand and sharing relevant facts with each other so that everyone is on the same page (AHRQ, 2019). Mutual support is the anticipation of team members' needs and shifting of workload to achieve balance during periods of high workload or stress (Health Research & Educational Trust, 2015). Interprofessional teams that perform with an understanding of each member's roles and responsibilities, both as individuals and as members of the team, contribute to a culture of quality and safety (King et al., 2008). This level of team effectiveness requires mutual trust, adaptability, open communication, and shared goals (Birnback & Salas, 2020; Frankel et al., 2017). TeamSTEPPS© tools and strategies utilized by nurses on interprofessional teams have been shown to facilitate structured team communication (Buljac-Samardzic et al., 2020; Krivanek et al., 2020). Standardized communication methods such as SBAR (situation, background, assessment, recommendations), team briefs and huddles, hand-offs, and debriefing checklists reduce the barriers to effective communication (Frankel et al., 2017; Lee et al., 2020). For more on how to use these communication methods see Chapter 3. Transparent communication and timely feedback, shared in a respectful and timely manner, contributes to a team and organizational culture that strives for continuous improvement (Armstrong, 2019). As leaders and change agents, nurses can advocate for adoption of these strategies, as well as organizational support for continued team training.

Sub-Competency 6.2d: Recognize How One's Uniqueness (as a Person and a Nurse) Contributes to Effective Interprofessional Working Relationships

SCENARIO 2

Mrs. Rios, a 68-year-old patient admitted with an exacerbation of chronic obstructive pulmonary disease, tells Tina, her registered nurse, "I just don't feel right this morning; not sure why. I just feel like something bad's about to happen." Tina has been Ms. Rios's nurse for the past 3 days, and other than subtle changes in her vital signs and the patient's anxiety, doesn't identify any other changes in her condition during the morning health assessment. Tina mentions the interaction to another staff nurse, who tells her to just "wait and watch" to see if anything changes. Tina is unsure but grows increasingly concerned for her patient and so decides to call the rapid response team to further evaluate Mrs. Rios. The team, composed of a physician, an ICU registered nurse, and a respiratory therapist, responds to the call.

Discussion Questions

1. Tina uses SBAR-R to communicate her concerns to the team. Outline the information Tina would use during her report to the team.
2. With minimal overt signs of a change in condition, was Tina right to call in the rapid response team or should she have waited, as suggested by the staff nurse? Why or why not?
3. What knowledge, skills, and attitudes (KSAs) do the members of the rapid response team need to possess to be effective in this situation?
4. What TeamSTEPPS or other approaches can the members of the rapid response team use to successfully incorporate Tina and Mrs. Rios into their time-limited team structure?

Team performance is also described in the Sunnybrook competency framework (McLaney et al., 2022). This framework specifically addresses interprofessional collaboration (Figure 4.2). In this framework, collaboration: (a) clinical and professional practice and care, (b) education, (c) research and quality improvement, and (d) approach to leadership (McLaney et al., 2022, p. 113). Interprofessional care is defined as "working together to deliver the highest quality of care," and interprofessional education is "defined as learning about, from and with each other" (p. 113). Interprofessional research and quality improvement entails two or more professions coming together to "integrate expertise and scientific perspectives to answer a shared research question or address a quality issue" (McLaney et al., 2022, p. 114). Interprofessional leadership includes "drawing on the strengths and capacities of team members in all professions and roles" (p. 114). Importantly, according to the Sunnybrook framework, interprofessional leadership "recognizes the importance of multiple voices and perspectives to achieve organizational and cultural change in an environment of complexity" (McLaney et al., 2022, p. 114).

The AHRQ distinguishes leaders as designated or situational. A designated leader is the person assigned to lead and organize a team, while a situational leader is any team member who has the skills to manage the specific situation (AHRQ, 2018b). Consider the example of a comprehensive care team for type 1 diabetes management. The endocrinologist, or an endocrinology nurse practitioner, might be the designated leader. However, if the patient's condition is found to be poorly controlled because of difficulty meal planning, the dietician may be the situational leader in helping the team and the family to improve outcomes. Or if the primary deficit is in the family's understanding of the nature of diabetes care, the nurse educator might situationally lead the team and the family toward implementation of a more successful comprehensive care plan. The fluid nature of leadership and expertise in the Sunnybrook model depicts this concept of designated versus situational leadership (Mc-Laney et al., 2018).

Leadership is the "glue" that holds a teamwork system together (AHRQ, 2018b). The leader ensures that the plan is conveyed to all team members, is continuously reviewed, and is updated as needed (AHRQ, 2018b). Any changes to the plan of action need to be relayed to the members of the team in a timely and direct manner. The RN in the team leader role can provide task assistance, assure balanced workload within the team, and model effective team behaviors (AHRQ, 2018b). Requirements for this leadership include communication, continuous monitoring, and fostering an environment of mutual support (AHRQ, 2018b). Bittner (2018) compares the role of the nurse as team leader to that of an air traffic controller, being intimately familiar with

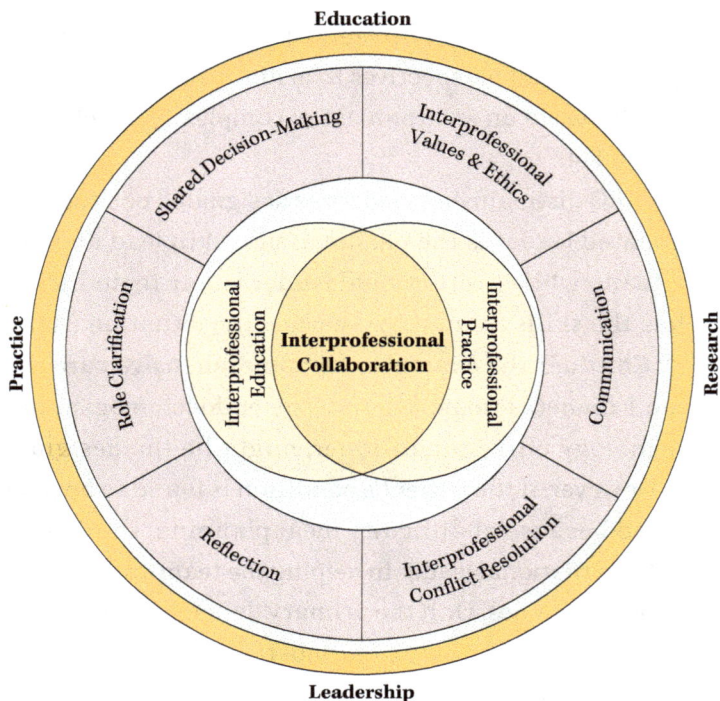

FIGURE 4.2   Sunnybrook interprofessional collaboration framework.

the clinical situation, but also having a clear understanding of each team member's roles and responsibilities within their scope of practice.

At the height of practice authority, an APRN, in particular, is in a position for designated leadership of an interprofessional team to develop a comprehensive plan of care as noted in AACN competency 2.5h. The degree to which an APRN is permitted to formally lead a plan of care or an interprofessional team may be based in part on state license or institutional parameters or restrictions. The consensus model was developed by the Advanced Practice Nursing Consensus Work Group and the National Council of State Boards of Nursing (NCSBN, 2023)

APRN Committee in order to "[provide] guidance for states to adopt uniformity in the regulation of APRN roles, licensure, accreditation, certification and education" (para. 1). As of October 2022, 27 of the states in the United States permit full practice authority, meaning that state practice and licensure laws permit nurse practitioners (NPs) to perform all elements within the scope of their practice under the exclusive licensure authority of the state board of nursing (AANP, 2022). Of note, this model is recommended by the National Academy of Medicine and the National Council of State Boards of Nursing (AANP, 2022). Alternately, 13 states have reduced practice, whereby state practice and licensure laws reduce the ability of the APRN to engage in at least one element of NP practice (AANP, 2022). One example of restriction is a career-long regulated collaborative agreement with another health provider in order to provide patient care. According to an AACN, a collaborative practice agreement is "a written statement that defines the joint practice of a physician and an APN [APRN] in a collaborative and complementary working relationship. It provides a mechanism for the legal protection of the APN [APRN] and sets out the rights and responsibilities of each party involved" (Herman & Ziel, 1999, p. 338). Under the agreement, cooperation among persons with complementary roles have shared responsibility for carrying out patient care plans with a recognition of the knowledge and skills of other team members. However, particularly in the case of restricted practice, supervision imposes an element of power differential that is not inherent interprofessional collaboration. Restricted autonomy may result in an APRN questioning one's expertise. Currently, 11 U.S. states have restricted practice, whereby state practice and licensure restrict the ability of an APRN to engage in at least one element of practice, typically requiring career-long supervision, delegation, or team management by another health provider (AANP, 2022).

Sub-Competency 6.2i: Reflect on How One's Role and Expertise Influences Team Performance

Sub-Competency 2.5h: Lead and Collaborate With an Interprofessional Team to Develop a Comprehensive Plan of Care

SCENARIO 3

Following the COVID-19 pandemic, many schools in the United States began to recognize negative behavioral and educational patterns in their student populations. In one urban area in a southeastern state, the public school system declared a child and adolescent mental health crisis. They reached out to their local large children's hospital for assistance and support. The children's hospital assessed its pediatric resources and realized that it did not have sufficient child psychiatrists or psychiatric NPs to provide individual care to each child in need. However, they employed a primary care pediatric nurse practitioner (PNP) who had recently relocated from a full-practice authority state, where for the past 15 years she managed a robust panel of children and adolescents needing treatment for mental health conditions such as attention-deficit/hyperactivity disorder (ADHD), depression, and anxiety. In that role, she regularly collaborated with other mental health professionals, as she typically diagnosed and prescribed medications, and they provided therapy and other support services. She was approached by the children's hospital to develop an interprofessional team consisting of a psychiatrist, a pediatrician, herself as the PNP, a child psychologist, and two social workers in order to develop comprehensive plans of care for these students.

The PNP was eager to lead the interprofessional team, given her expertise in child and adolescent mental health and enthusiasm for collaboration. However, she soon learned that due to the restricted practice nature of this state, she was not permitted to prescribe any psychiatric medications to patients under 18 years of age, since she was not licensed as a psychiatric nurse. She presented her background to the credentialing committee, noting that her PNP curriculum extensively addressed pediatric mental health care and that she had attended several conferences and completed multiple continuing education modules specifically addressing pediatric mental health care. She discussed her 15 years of experience prescribing medications such as selective serotonin reuptake inhibitors (SSRIs), selective norepinephrine reuptake inhibitors (SNRIs), and stimulant medications for ADHD, with strong evidence of positive results. She shared her passion for collaboration with the mental health care community. Ultimately, the credentialing committee declined to position her as leader of the interprofessional team, citing state restrictions hindering her ability to perform in this capacity. They welcomed her to participate on the team, as long as she discussed every student's case with the psychiatrist on the team, who was planning to continue her own robust private practice with a 3-month waitlist for appointments.

Discussion Questions

1. In this scenario, what is the impact of role restrictions on the APRN's practice in
    the interprofessional team
    the comprehensive plan of care
    the patient population?
2. How would you advise that the PNP respond to the credentialing committee and the interprofessional team?
3. Describe strategies nurses can employ to advocate for increased autonomy as appropriate for their role on an interprofessional team.

Development of Expertise

Nurses at entry- and advanced-practice levels are encouraged to pursue the full scope of their practice as a means of gaining expertise. The development of expertise in nursing has been well described by Benner (1984, 2001). Benner's model describes the nurse as passing through five stages of professional development: novice, advanced beginner, competent, proficient, and expert. Transition from novice to proficient is thought to take between 3 and 5 years, with an additional 5 years to become an expert (Benner, 2001). Similarly, Brown and Olshansky (1997) described the transition to the NP role. In examining the experiences of recently graduated NPs during their first year of primary care practice, this model consists of a process called "from limbo to legitimacy" (Brown & Olshansky, 1997). The four major categories are laying the foundation, launching, meeting the challenge, and broadening the perspective (Brown & Olshansky, 1997). These categories are not necessarily linear or mutually exclusive. A newly graduated APRN may be described as "in limbo" when they hold the academic credentials but not the license or employment to practice as an NP (Huffstutler & Varnell, 2006).

Even an RN or advanced-level nurse with established expertise may perceive that their accomplishments are inadequate or false, compromising their role performance on the team. This is well described by a concept known as *imposter phenomenon* or *imposter syndrome*. First described by Pauline Clance and Suzanne Imes in 1978, it was shown to be more prevalent among women and particularly women of color (Psychology Today, 2023). It has now evolved to a broader understanding of how successful persons feel like frauds. Imposter syndrome is known to be associated with personality traits, such as perfectionism and diminished self-efficacy; competitive environments; and high-pressure/achievement-oriented upbringing as children (Psychology Today, 2023). Nurses may be particularly vulnerable to experiencing imposter syndrome due to the rigorous and competitive nature of nursing school, coupled with the well-respected profession that they enter, and amplified by high-stress and mentally and physically demanding roles (Falcone, 2023). It is not uncommon for new nurses to report feeling unworthy, unprepared, or incapable (Falcone, 2023). APRNs are expected to achieve even higher levels of expertise and may therefore be at increased risk. Studies among CRNAs, CNSs, and FNPs have validated this finding (Darna, 2022; Haney et al., 2018; Heitz et al., 2004). In a qualitative study of recently graduated family nurse practitioners (FNPs; Heitz et al., 2004), optimistic self-talk with comments such as "you've got to keep working" and "you're prepared to do this" served as a coping mechanism during what is often a difficult transition period. Positive self-talk in times of uncertainty is a great example of AACN competency 6.2i: "Reflect on how one's role and expertise influences team performance." According to Huffstutler and Varnell (2006), "The NP who engages in self-reflection, the act of calmly looking inward or giving attentive meditation to a subject, will work through the transitional process more effectively, as opposed to spending time on fears or denying one's limitations" (p. 12). In a workshop for addressing the impacts of imposter syndrome on clinical nurse specialists, Haney et al. (2018) recommended these specific strategies: giving the feeling a name; identifying and talking to a mentor for realistic feedback; remembering what they do well; realizing that no one is perfect; and practicing thought-stopping strategies. According to Kaiser Permanente (2022), thought stopping is a technique to help you stop unwanted thoughts in order to help you change your feelings about them.

Sub-Competency 6.2i Reflect on How One's Role and Expertise Influences Team Performance

Consider your past or ideal experience on an interprofessional team.

1. When did I feel qualified or valued as a member of an interprofessional team?
2. What was my expertise on that team?
3. What is an area of strength that I brought to my team?
4. How does my uniqueness (as a person and a nurse) contribute to effective interprofessional working relationships?

CONCLUSION

Health care providers and organizations have acknowledged the value of effective interprofessional teams as they relate to improved patient safety, satisfaction, and health outcomes.

Concerted time, effort, and commitment goes into creating and supporting effective interprofessional teams. Unfortunately, educational and psychological barriers prevent effective team performance. Few health care providers have the opportunity to receive interprofessional training in teamwork and communication during their education (Zajac et al., 2021). Most training programs focus on discipline-specific roles and responsibilities with little meaningful interaction with individuals in other professional groups. Power and hierarchical structures further limit team performance (Weller et al., 2014). Health professional students often are socialized to believe team leadership is limited to those with more advanced academic degrees or clinical experience. This misconception can be reinforced in clinical settings where there is little exposure to effective interprofessional teams. The result is team members feeling they are only capable of playing a supporting role on the team and that their input has limited value. Increasing opportunities for health care professionals from different backgrounds and disciplines to work in teams can lead to a more comprehensive understanding of each provider's roles and responsibilities, as individuals and as members of an interprofessional team (Interprofessional Education Collaborative Expert Panel, 2011). These interactions, along with structured learning activities and self-reflection, can promote greater appreciation of the contributions of each team member, leading to increased civility, respect (Furr et al., 2020), and a "more positive, engaging, and resilient workplace" (Rosen et al., 2018, p. xx). Effective team performance contributes to improved communication, collaboration, and ultimately improved health outcomes for patients and their families (Frankel et al., 2017; Rosen et al., 2018).

KEY POINTS

- Effective teamwork requires collaboration, in which persons with complementary roles cooperatively work together toward a common goal.
- Team dynamics describe how a team communicates, interacts, and works together and are a major influence on the effectiveness of a team.
- Team roles are the responsibilities assigned to or associated with a person's position on a team and may be based on competencies, expertise, or designation.
- Competency is a measure of capability to perform successfully and can be evaluated from an individual or team perspective.
- Expertise describes expert knowledge or skill in a particular subject, activity, or job. Expertise within a team may be fluid, variable, and situation specific and is not always directly related to clinical expertise.
- Just culture describes an environment of civility and respect in which errors are addressed from a nonblaming standpoint, which improves safety and reliability within interprofessional teams.
- Leadership is the glue that holds a team together and includes oversight, communication, and revision of the team plan as indicated. All nurses can provide leadership on interprofessional teams, and an APRN is particularly suited to designated leadership of the comprehensive plan of care.

ACTIVITIES

Activity 1: Exploring Team Communication Strategies
Using the TeamSTEPPS© pocket guide, https://www.ahrq.gov/teamstepps-program/resources/pocket-guide/index.html,

imagine a scenario in which you could use the communication strategies listed. Work alone or with a partner to practice each strategy.

1. call-out

2. check-back

3. hand-off

4. "I pass the baton"

Activity 2: Self-Reflection: Imagine Yourself ...

Consider the topics discussed in this chapter, as they relate to your role as a nurse:

1. What do you feel you're doing well as a member of the health care team?

2. What improvements can you make to your team role performance?

3. Do you think that your performance on the team will change after graduation or licensing? If so, how?

4. What do you envision as your team role after 5 years in your nursing practice?

Activity 3: "Thought-Stopping" Exercise

Imagine a situation in which stressful thoughts might occur (i.e., questioning your role on the team or your level of expertise), and then do the following:

- Practice closing your eyes, taking a deep breath, and saying stop, either aloud or internally.
- Replace an unwanted thought with a more pleasant or inspiring thought or image, such as envisioning yourself successfully leading a team.

- Snap your fingers whenever unpleasant thoughts enter your mind, both as a distraction from the thought and as a reminder to consider what may be triggering those thoughts.

REFERENCES

Accreditation Council for Continuing Medical Education. (2021). *FAQs.* https://www.accme.org/faq/what-interprofessional-team-described-engages-teams-criterion

Agency for Healthcare Research and Quality. (2018a). *TeamSTEPPS© fundamentals course: Module 2. Team structure.* https://www.ahrq.gov/teamstepps/instructor/fundamentals/module2/slteamstruct.html

Agency for Healthcare Research and Quality. (2018b). *TeamSTEPPS© fundamentals course: Module 4. Leading teams.* https://www.ahrq.gov/teamstepps/instructor/fundamentals/module4/slleadership.html#im1

Agency for Healthcare Research and Quality. (2019). *TeamSTEPPS© fundamentals course: Module 5. Situation monitoring.* https://www.ahrq.gov/teamstepps/instructor/fundamentals/module5/igsitmonitor.html

American Association of Colleges of Nursing (2021). *The Essentials: Core Competencies for Professional Nursing Education.* pp. 29–32. https://www.aacnnursing.org/Portals/0/PDFs/Publications/Essentials-2021.pdf

American Association of Nurse Practitioners. (2022). *State practice environment.* https://www.aanp.org/advocacy/state/state-practice-environment?gclid=Cj0KCQiAxbefBhDfARIsAL4XLRqUHVQrlyaKRXu1h3O-h30Aq7_vHomevkPhcGbZI2JhXgPWPgqQFHykaAmzvEALw_wcB

American Nurses Association. (2015). *Nursing: Scope and standards of practice* (3rd ed.).

Armstrong, G. (2019). QSEN safety competency: The key ingredient is just culture. *Journal of Continuing Education in Nursing, 50(*10), 444–447. https://doi.org/10.3928/00220124-20190917-05

Balmer, J. (2020). Nursing professional development practitioners in leadership roles. *Journal for Nurses in Professional Development, 36*(3)167–169. https://www.doi.org/10.1097/NND.0000000000000626

Belker, L., McCormick, J., & Topchik, G. (2019). *Team dynamics.* American Management Association. https://www.amanet.org/articles/team-dynamics/

Benner, P. (1982). From novice to expert. *AJN The American Journal of Nursing, 82*(3), 402–407.

Benner, P. (2001). *From novice to expert: Excellence and power in clinical nursing practice.* Commemorative Edition, Prentice Hall, Upper Saddle River.

Birnback, D., & Salas, E. (2020). Patient safety and team training. In D. H. Chestnut, C. A. Wong, L. C Tsen, W. D Ngan Kee, Y. Beilin, J. Mhyre, B.T. Bateman, & N. Nathan (Eds.), *Chestnut's obstetric anesthesia: Principles and practice* (6th ed., chapter 11).

Bittner, C. A. (2018). The importance of role clarity for development of interprofessional teams. *Journal of Continuing Education in Nursing, 49*(8), 345–347.

Brown, M. A., & Olshansky, E. F. (1997). From limbo to legitimacy: A theoretical model of the transition to the primary care nurse practitioner role. *Nursing Research., 46*(1), 46–51. https://doi.org/10.1097/00006199-199701000-00008

Buljac-Samardzic, M., Doekhie, K., & van Wijngaarden, J. (2020). Interventions to improve team effectiveness within health care: A systematic review of the past decade. *Human Resources for Health, 18*(2), 1–42. https://doi.org/10.1186/s12960-019-0411-3

Collins English Dictionary (2023) https://www.collinsdictionary.com/us/.

Committee on Measuring the Impact of Interprofessional Education on Collaborative Practice and Patient Outcomes; Board on Global Health; Institute of Medicine. (2015). Measuring the impact of interprofessional education on collaborative practice and patient outcomes. Washington (DC): National Academies Press (US). Available from: https://www.ncbi.nlm.nih.gov/books/NBK338360/ doi: 10.17226/21726

Darna, J. R. (2022). *A description of impostor phenomenon in certified registered nurse anesthesiologists* (no. 919). Doctoral dissertation, University of San Diego. https://doi.org/10.22371/07.2022.001

Dingel, H., Wager, E., McGough, M., Rakshit, S., Telesford, I., Schwartz, H., Cox, C., & Amin, K. (n.d.). *The state of the U.S. health system in 2022 and the outlook for 2023.* Health System Tracker. https://www.healthsystemtracker.org/brief/the-state-of-the-u-s-health-system-in-2022-and-the-outlook-for-2023/#Total%20deaths%20in%20the%20United%20States%20from%20COVID-19%20and%20other%20leading%20causes,%20 2020-2022

Falcone, S. (2023, July 21). *3 tips to overcome imposter syndrome as a nurse.* Nurse.org. https://nurse.org/articles/nurse-imposter-syndrome/#:~:text=Imposter%20Syndrome%2C%20or%20impostorism%2C%20 refers,causes%20debilitating%20anxiety%20and%20depression

Frankel, A., Haraden, C., Federico, F, & Lenoci-Edwards, J. (2017). *A framework for safe, reliable, and effective care* [White Paper]. Institute for Healthcare Improvement and Safe and Reliable Healthcare.

Furr, S., Lane, S., Martin, D., & Brackney, D. (2020). Understanding roles in health care through interprofessional educational experiences. *British Journal of Nursing, 29*(6), 364–372.

Haney, T. S., Birkholz, L., & Rutledge, C. (2018). A workshop for addressing the impact of the imposter syndrome on clinical nurse specialists.

Clinical Nurse Specialist, 32(4), 189–194. https://doi.org/10.1097/nur.0000000000000386

Harper, M., Warren, J., Bradley, D., Bindon, S., & Maloney, P. (2019). Nursing professional development's spirit of inquiry focus areas. *Journal for Nurses in Professional Development, 35*(3), 118–124. https://doi.org/10.1097/NND.0000000000000515

Health Quality Council of Alberta. (2023). *What is a just culture?* https://justculture.hqca.ca/what-is-a-just-culture/#:~:text=A%20just%20culture%20is%20a%20small%20part%20of,wrong%20or%20nearly%20goes%20wrong%20with%20patient%20care

Health Research & Educational Trust. (2015, June). *Improving patient safety culture through teamwork and communication: TeamSTEPPS®.* https://psnet.ahrq.gov/issue/improving-patient-safety-culture-through-teamwork-and-communication-teamstepps

Heitz, L. J., Steiner, S. H., & Burman, M. E. (2004). RN to FNP: A qualitative study of role transition. *The Journal of Nursing Education, 43*(9), 416–420. https://doi.org/10.3928/01484834-20040901-08

Herman, J., & Ziel, S. (1999). Collaborative practice agreements for advanced practice nurses: What you should know. *AACN Clinical Issues, 10*(3), 337–342. https://doi.org/10.1097/00044067-199908000-00003

Huffstutler, S. Y., & Varnell, G. (2006, June 7). *The impostor phenomenon: New NPS.* Medscape. https://www.medscape.com/viewarticle/533648

Interprofessional Education Collaborative Expert Panel. (2011). *Core competencies for interprofessional collaborative practice: Report of an expert panel.* Interprofessional Education Collaborative.

Kaiser Permanente. (2022). *Stop negative thoughts: Getting started.* https://healthy.kaiserpermanente.org/health-wellness/health-encyclopedia/he.stop-negative-thoughts-getting-started.uf9938

King, H. B., Battles, J., Baker, D. P., Alonso, A., Salas, E., Webster, J., Toomey, L., & Salisbury, M. (2008). *TeamSTEPPS®: Team strategies and tools to enhance performance and patient safety.* https://www.ncbi.nlm.nih.gov/books/NBK43686/

Koehne, K. (2018). Nurturing a spirit of inquiry. *American Academy of Ambulatory Care Nursing, 40*(4), 20–21.

Krivanek, M., Dolansky, M., Goliat, L., & Petty, G. (2020). Implementing TeamSTEPPS® to facilitate workplace civility and nurse retention. *Journal for Nurses in Professional Development, 36*(5), 259–265. https://doi.org/10.1097/NND.0000000000000666

Lee, K. R., & Kim, E. J. (2020). Relationship between interprofessional communication and team task performance. *Clinical Simulation in Nursing, 43*, 44–50. https://doi.org/10.1016/j.ecns.2020.02.002

Melnyk, B., Fineout-Overholt, E., Stillwell, S., & Williamson, K. (2009). Igniting a spirit of inquiry: An essential foundation for evidence-based practice. *American Journal of Nursing, 109*(11), 49–52.

McLaney, E., Morassaei, S., Hughes, L., Davies, R., Campbell, M., & Di Prospero, L. (2022). A framework for interprofessional team collaboration in a hospital setting: Advancing team competencies and behaviors. *Healthcare Management Forum, 35*(2), 112–117. https://doi.org/10.1177/08404704211063584

National Academies of Sciences, Engineering, and Medicine. (2011). *The future of nursing: Leading change, advancing health.* The National Academies Press. https://doi.org/10.17226/12956.

National Academies of Sciences, Engineering, and Medicine. (2021). T*he future of nursing 2020–2030: Charting a path to achieve health equity.* The National Academies Press. https://doi.org/10.17226/25982

National Council of State Boards of Nursing. (2023). *APRN campaign for consensus.* https://www.ncsbn.org/nursing-regulation/practice/aprn/aprn-consensus.page

O'Daniel, M. & Rosenstein, A.H. (2008). Professional communication and team collaboration. In: R.G. Hughes (Ed.), *Patient safety and quality: An evidence-based handbook for nurses.* Rockville (MD): Agency for Healthcare Research and Quality (US). Chapter 33. Available from: https://www.ncbi.nlm.nih.gov/books/NBK2637/

O'Donovan, R., & McAuliffe, E. (2020). Exploring psychological safety in healthcare teams to inform the development of interventions: combining observational, survey and interview data. *BMC Health Services Research, 20*(810), 1–16. https://doi.org/10.1186/s12913-020-05646-z.

Oxford Advanced Learner's Dictionary. (2023). *Expertise.* https://www.oxford-learnersdictionaries.com/us/definition/english/expertise?q=expertise

Paradiso, L., & Sweeney, N. (2019). Just culture: It's more than policy. *Nursing Management*, 39–45.

Psychology Today. (2023). *Imposter syndrome.* https://www.psychologytoday.com/us/basics/imposter-syndrome

Rosen, M., DiazGranados, D., Dietz, A., Benishek, L., Thompson, D., Pronovost, P., & Weaver, S. (2018). Teamwork in healthcare: Key discoveries enabling safer, high-quality care. *Am Psychol, 73*(4), 433–450. https://doi.org/10.1037/amp0000298

TeamSTEPPS Pocket Guide. Content last reviewed August 2023. Agency for Healthcare Research and Quality, Rockville, MD. https://www.ahrq.gov/teamstepps-program/resources/pocket-guide/index.html

Theodorou, M. E., Henschen, B. L., & Chapman, M. (2020). The comprehensive care plan: A patient-centered, multidisciplinary communication tool for frequently hospitalized patients. *The Joint Commission Journal on Quality and Patient Safety, 46*(4), 217–226. https://doi.org/10.1016/j.jcjq.2020.01.002.

von der Lancken, S., & Gunn, E. (2018). Improving role identity by shadowing interprofessional team members in a clinical setting: An innovative clinical education course. *Journal of Interprofessional Care*, *33*(5), 464–471. https://doi.org/10.1080/13561820.2018.1538940.

Weller, J., Boyde, M., & Cumin, D. (2014). Team, tribes and patient safety: Overcoming barriers to effective teamwork in healthcare. *Postgrad Medical Journal*, *90*, 149–154. https://doi.org/10.1136/postgradmedj-2012-131168

Zajac, S., Woods, A., Tannenbaum, S., Salas, E., & Holladay, C. (2021). Overcoming challenges to teamwork in healthcare: A team effectiveness framework and evidence-based guidance. *Frontiers in Communication*, *6*, 606445. https://doi.org/10.3389/fcomm.2021.606445

CREDITS

CHAPTER 5

Roles and Responsibilities

Marie D. Grosh, DNP, APRN-CNP, LNHA, Carli A. Carnish, DNP, RN, APRN-CNP, and Carol Savrin, DNP, CPNP, R, CNP-BC, FAANP, FNAP

KEY AACN COMPETENCIES, SUB-COMPETENCIES, AND CONCEPTS

Domain 6: Interprofessional Partnerships

Competency 6.2 Perform effectively in different team roles, using principles and values of team dynamics.

- *Advanced-Level Sub-Competency 6.2j* Foster positive team dynamics to strengthen desired outcomes.

Competency 6.3 Use knowledge of nursing and other professions to address health care needs.

- *Entry-Level Sub-Competency 6.3b* Leverage roles and abilities of team members to optimize care.
- *Entry-Level Sub-Competency 6.3c* Communicate with team members to clarify responsibilities in executing plan of care.

Domain 9: Professionalism

Competency 9.3 Demonstrate accountability to the individual, society, and the profession.

- *Advanced-Level Sub-Competency 9.3j* Demonstrate leadership skills when participating in professional activities and/or organizations.

Continued

Continued

Concepts for Nursing Practice

- Communication
- Evidence-based practice

KEY TERMS

Advocacy	Elaborative behavior
Collaboration	Partnerships
Cultural awareness	Professional identity
Delegation	Team dynamics
Diversity	Cognitive flexibility
Professional diversity	

INTRODUCTION: INTERPROFESSIONAL COMMUNICATION

Patient care is provided in a positive and productive way when there is effective communication and collaboration between members of an interprofessional team. Interprofessional teamwork has gained momentum as a critical approach to patient care due to rising patient complexity related to multimorbidity and health disparities of an increasingly diverse patient population. This has become exceedingly challenging, exacerbated by the COVID-19 pandemic and its sequelae. The benefits of interprofessional teamwork are multifactorial. Interprofessional collaboration can reduce the fragmentation that occurs in the U.S. health care system and provides opportunities to improve the efficiency and quality of care delivered while reducing overall costs.

Health care professionals from different professions bring different skills and different knowledge bases to patient care. The pharmacist has an in-depth knowledge of the medications that a patient is taking, while the physician has an in-depth knowledge of the disease entities that a patient has, and the nurse understands how the timing of the medications impacts life style and is impacted by the patient's disease entities. If all these health care professionals work together, they will have a greater ability to provide patient care that is not only comprehensive and compassionate but is simultaneously agreeable to the patient so that the long-term outcome is improved.

Be aware that it is not enough to just convene many different professions onto a team and expect better outcomes. Discerning each member's roles and responsibilities—including our own—is the first step in realizing the benefits of a professionally diverse team. Without a firm grasp of the topic, team members run the risk of operation in silos versus creating synergy. As discussed, if all the health care professionals do not talk to each other, the medications may not be timed correctly, and the medications might not be the most appropriate considering all the patient's disease entities. A deep understanding of team concepts and collaboration is the foundation on which to build complex workflows and communication systems for clinical success.

In 2011, the Interprofessional Education Collaborative (IPEC) released the original Core Competencies for Interprofessional Collaborative Practice. Competency domain 2 describes the professional roles and responsibilities of interprofessional team members. Updates to the original core competencies were published in 2016 with increased attention to population health and the patient experience. The defining attribute of competency domain 2, according to the IPEC, is "the use of one's own role and those of other professions to appropriately assess and address the health care needs of patients and to promote and advance the health of populations" (IPEC, 2016, p. 13, para. 2). Domain 2 sub-competencies are listed in Table 5.1. The American Association of Colleges of Nursing Essentials (AACN, 2021) provides defining features of the interprofessional team member roles and responsibilities for both entry- and advanced practice-level nurses under the competency domains of interprofessional partnerships and professionalism.

TABLE 5.1   Core Competencies for Interprofessional Collaborative Practice: Competency Domain 2—Roles/Responsibilities

Communicate one's roles and responsibilities clearly to patients, families, community members, and other professionals.
Recognize one's own limitations in skills, knowledge, and abilities.
Engage diverse professionals who complement one's own professional expertise, as well as associated resources, to develop strategies to meet specific health and health care needs of patients and populations.
Explain the roles and responsibilities of other care providers and how the teams work together to provide care, promote health, and prevent disease.
Use the full scope of knowledge, skills, and abilities of professionals from health and other fields to provide care that is safe, timely, efficient, effective, and equitable.
Communicate with team members to clarify each member's responsibility in executing components of a treatment plan or public health intervention.
Forge independent relationships with other professions within and outside of the health system to improve care and advance learning.
Engage in continuous professional and interprofessional development to enhance team performance and collaboration.
Use the unique and complementary abilities of all members of the team to optimize health and patient care.
Describe how professionals in health and other fields can collaborate and integrate clinical care and public health interventions to optimize patient health.

Nurses, integral members of the interprofessional team, often serve as the coordinator of patient care. Nurses are well equipped to perform the role of team leader, manager, or care coordinator, as holistic patient-centered care is a core feature of nursing practice. Care coordination between physicians, advanced-practice providers, unlicensed medical personnel, and other health care providers most often is the nurse's responsibility in their regular day-to-day clinical practice. It is generally the nurse who is available to communicate with the unlicensed personnel who perhaps did the bed bath and noticed the beginning of a pressure ulcer, and the nurse then can communicate that to the physical therapist and the physician. The nurse needs to recognize that they are often the center of the wheel when coordination of care is required. Nurses need to feel empowered to speak up in interprofessional situations.

APPLICATION TO PRACTICE

Professional Identity

A solid sense of one's own professional identity is an important quality of each role in the interprofessional team. Nurses must recognize that their role brings a perspective that is unique and relevant to contribute. If the nurse can identify and effectively communicate what professional knowledge and skills their discipline has to offer, the potential for successful teamwork and patient care outcomes rises significantly. This increases the likelihood that team communication will be bidirectional and not solely focused on a single patient problem. As the caregiver with most frequent contact, the nursing role is often more familiar with the unique and complex needs of the patient and family. Nurses can help to identify both functional and learning needs in addition to potential barriers and/or facilitators to a successful plan of care. The nurse should also show appreciation and respect for the expertise and contributions from other team members.

Alternatively, this may result in a dilemma for novice or advanced-beginner nurses as they are still developing and honing their skills. A less experienced nurse may lack confidence and feel intimidated working with other members of the interprofessional team. This can negatively impact their likelihood to offer input and participate within the team to their fullest potential. When one member does not participate in a team effort, the patient outcome can be negatively impacted.

Entry-Level Sub-Competency 6.3c: Communicate With Team Members to Clarify Responsibilities in Executing Plan of Care

SCENARIO 1

Sally Smith is a new graduate nurse on a cardiac stepdown unit who has just completed the new hire orientation period. Today is her first shift working independently without her nurse coach. Her unit recently implemented a nurse-led interdisciplinary team rounding initiative, and she is expected to participate. The cardiothoracic surgeon, nurse practitioner, pharmacist, and social worker arrive at the unit for rounds just after Sally has finished receiving report from the night shift RN. Sally's first patient on rounds is a 50-year-old male who is postoperative day 2 following a four-vessel coronary artery bypass graft surgery. He was transferred from the cardiac intensive-care unit early this morning, just 2 hours before shift change. The night shift RN's handoff report on this patient to Sally this morning was very brief, telling Sally, "I don't know much about him; he just got here." Apparently last night, the patient went into atrial fibrillation with rapid ventricular response. The surgical house coverage physician ordered him a loading dose of digoxin and intravenous heparin. Unfortunately, this information was not conveyed to Sally during the report, nor was the primary surgical team notified. As the pharmacist reviewed the patient's list of medications, he asked Sally why the patient was receiving these medications and when they were started. Sally searches through the patient's electronic health record to answer his questions, but the surgeon becomes impatient and loudly yells at Sally, "How could you not know why this patient is taking these drugs, and why wasn't I notified of this? What kind of nurse are you?" Flustered, Sally apologizes and eventually provides the information requested.

Discussion Questions

1. How might this interaction impact the other members of the inter-professional team?
2. How might this interaction impact the nurse–patient relationship?
3. Was there a breakdown in role on someone's part?
4. Who or how will this be communicated to the night nurse in a respectful manner?
5. How might this interaction impact the culture and climate of the cardiac stepdown unit?
6. Identify key opportunities to improve care in this scenario.
7. Identify strategies for improvement for the patient, team, and institution.

Cognitive Flexibility

Recognizing one's own value and contributions are only one role of the nurse in interprofessional teamwork. To meet the AACN's competency standards, the nurse must also develop and exhibit cognitive flexibility. The AACN (2021) describes cognitive flexibility as "the ability to adapt flexibly to a constantly changing environment" (p. 56). Cognitive flexibility allows the nurse to multitask effectively; however, it is not an inherent skill (Koch et al., 2018). The makeup of each interprofessional team is unique and dependent on the needs of each patient or population, and therefore the nurse is expected to respond and adapt appropriately.

Exercising cognitive flexibility may be challenging for new entry- or advanced-level nurses who are still in an intense learning phase and have not had as much opportunity to develop this skill. Cognitive flexibility allows the individual to disengage from a previous task, engage in a new one, and accomplish that and then switch back (Dajani & Uddin, 2015). The new graduate often has difficulty with this switch. More seasoned nurses accomplish the switch more easily as they have often had experience with both tasks. The new graduate entry-level nurses often report feeling overwhelmed and may perceive themselves as burdens rather than assets to the interprofessional team (St Martin et al., 2015). Student nurses and new nurses should reflect on positive performance feedback from faculty and preceptors to realize their strengths and valuable contributions to interdisciplinary teams.

Advanced-Level Sub-Competency 6.2j: Cultivating Functional Team Dynamics

SCENARIO 2

Grant Weber, RN, is on the orthopedic floor. This is the first day that he will be on his own without his mentor to guide him. He has three patients, and they are all very similar to ones that he has been caring for during his orientation. He feels quite comfortable caring for these patients. He has his schedule worked out quite well and has all the meds and care activities organized. He is doing a dressing change on Mr. Garcia when Martha, one of the unlicensed personnel, comes and tells him that Mrs. Chen is acting very strange. She seems to be slurring her words and not making sense. Grant tells the Martha that he will be right there. He does not want to leave the dressing undone, so he proceeds to finish that task. Meanwhile, Martha is getting frustrated waiting and tells another RN about Mrs. Chen. When Grant gets into the room, the other RN has called the provider and thinks that Mrs. Chen had a stroke. The other RN is *very* upset with Grant for not coming immediately. The provider comes and, after some questioning of both Grant and the other RN, determines that Mrs. Chen is a diabetic and needs sugar. Now the provider is angry with both RNs for not knowing the patient history and not thinking about what might have happened. Grant feels terrible and decides that he is not cut out to work on his own.

Discussion Questions

1. How might Grant have handled the situation differently?
2. How might the other RN have handled the situation differently?
3. What might be a better way to deal with an interruption of one task for another?
4. How might Grant follow up with the provider?

Team Diversity, Equity, and Inclusion

Nurses must demonstrate cultural awareness and cultural competence. In nursing education, the terms *cultural awareness* and *cultural competence* are often used in describing the nurse's role working with patients or populations. While this is of course essential in providing patient-centered care, these behaviors are also required to facilitate communication and convey respect toward other team members. Nurses should also encourage other members of the interprofessional team to practice cultural awareness and familiarize themselves with the cultural context of others.

The diversity that exists in interprofessional teams is what contributes to their successful functioning. However, in health care there often is a hierarchical structure that inhibits certain team members from contributing as much as others. Team members may feel too intimidated to "speak up" when they see an existing or potential conflict. Power struggles are a major barrier to effective team performance and need to be recognized early on and rectified. Just as the nurse should not feel subservient to physicians or advanced-practice providers, neither should unlicensed medical or nursing personnel. As the nurse is often their primary point of contact, they should encourage these team members to participate in team discussions, offering information or suggestions. There are often situations in which the unlicensed personnel have more experience with a patient when bathing them or feeding them and may have very valuable information to share with the team. When each member of the team views their collaboration as a partnership, this promotes inclusion of all team members' ideas, resulting in a more effective patient-centered plan of care.

All health care team members need to learn to use inclusive language—language that makes people feel included. In health care, how we discuss and address people matters because everyone deserves to feel seen through the lens of equity, validated, and treated with respect and dignity. This applies to members of the team as well as patients. It also applies when discussing patients in and among team members. The nurse should use inclusive language when relating to patients and respectfully remind others to do so as well.

Team dynamics are the relationships and behaviors that influence the performance of a group. They can be considered functional when the goals of patient care are achieved and the team members are satisfied with the process. Successful teamwork does not come easily; problematic dynamics are often a challenge and can negatively impact quality and safety in patient care. Some literature estimates that over 70% of medical errors are attributable to dysfunctional team dynamics (Mitchell et al., 2014; Salas et al., 2017).

Fostering positive dynamics is a critical responsibility of the advanced-level nurse on an interprofessional team. This involves being aware of the main components of successful team dynamics, anticipating and identifying common barriers, and facilitating solutions. Key aspects of team dynamics that the advanced-level nurse must be aware of include professional diversity and identifications, cooperative goals, and elaborative behaviors (Mitchell et al., 2014). Team members need to have a sense of psychological safety in order to be willing to participate in team activities. If a team member does not feel safe in the situation, they may not be willing to speak up when needed. For more on psychological safety see Chapter 7

DIVERSITY AND ROLE IDENTIFICATIONS: FINDING THE RIGHT MIX

Professional diversity is the extent to which there are a variety of different professions and educational backgrounds represented in a team. However, the more diverse a team is, the more individual role identifications there are, which can sometimes have a negative impact on dynamics. This section will explore how role identifications within a diverse team of clinicians has a mediating effect on how professional diversity can help or hurt the team's success.

On one hand, greater professional diversity can provide a team with a broader range of knowledge, increasing the likelihood that one of the team members will hold the "solution" to a patient problem in their knowledge base. This is the magic that creates the synergistic positive outcomes of interprofessional teamwork by increasing efficiency and offering different perspectives. However, some research has purported a negative or no relationship between professional diversity and positive team outcomes. That seems counterintuitive, so how can that be? High degrees of strong, deeply held views and intense attachment and identification with one's profession often results in protection of professional knowledge as a source of power and identity (Fitzgerald & Teal, 2004). Individuals with strong professional identity are more profoundly driven by the priorities of their profession and more likely to feel threatened by pressure to accommodate alternative perspectives (Mitchell et al., 2014). Therefore, to capitalize on the asset pool of a diverse team, an advanced-level nurse should assess the level of professional identification of team members—including nursing (i.e., self-assessment)—to ensure that all members are open to participating in collaborative problem solving that involves an open exchange, discussion, and friendly debate of ideas.

This can begin by looking at educational backgrounds. Identification is encouraged during each profession's education program at varying levels, and then internalized at varying degrees within individuals (AACN, 2021; Cruess et al., 2014). If you are not familiar with the role of a team member, visit the website of the profession's certifying body and read about the educational background and other requirements. Use these as conversation starters to discern specific details (e.g., "I have read that PAs earn various medical degrees before beginning their PA program. What was your first degree in?"). Remember that roles and responsibilities often differ between organizations and situations. For example, in one setting a physician on a team may be responsible for direct care and in another may play only a consultative role or a supervisory/quality improvement role. Obtaining clear information about the organization's assigned responsibilities for a profession in addition to each member's personal identification with their role is important.

Next, ask questions of team members about their motivations: Why are they here? What are their goals? Answers that are profession focused ("I am here to represent the physical therapy team," "Each team needs a physician leader") versus patient outcome focused ("I am here to help prevent immobility during the patients' recovery") may elucidate areas in which the APRN can guide members toward a shared purpose that is patient centered. Discourage logistic motivations ("I am here because my manager told me to be") or motivations that are too general ("I am here to provide care"), as these can often be toxic or a sign of ambivalence.

Now think of your role in the team situation and answer the same questions for yourself. This exercise can be enlightening from the perspective of other team members but also helps you to understand your role in the situation. This helps you understand your role not only in relation to other team members but also related to the patient.

Do team members have any other commitments, whether personal or organizational, that will impact the team's work? What are the feelings about these commitments? These can often go unsaid, but it is important to establish a spirit of openness to avoid assumptions. Clinicians frequently feel uncomfortable sharing other commitments for fear of seeming unengaged. The APRN as a team leader could share one first, opening the conversation. For example, "Administration let me know they want me to discharge three patients by Friday to open up beds for the weekend. That is frustrating because I'm not sure I will be able to safely accomplish that." Then other team members may feel comfortable sharing, "The therapy team gets a bonus at the end of the month based on our readmission rates"; "The pharmacy has been tasked with reducing the number of BEERs (a list of medications that are inappropriate for elderly patients, first identified by Dr. Beers) criteria prescriptions by 10%"; or "I am planning to gather data on this team's outcomes to publish in a medical journal." In addition to the comfort of transparency, this activity creates a sense of trust and community in that we all have other pressures which can sometimes conflict and pull us in varying directions.

TABLE 5.2 **Role Identification Questions**

Professional identification: "Who are you?"	Motivations: "Why are *you* here?"	Shared problem definition and goals: "Why are *we* here?"

Critical Questions When Establishing Positive Team Dynamics

COOPERATIVE GOALS

Once motivations and commitments are established and role identifications of each profession are at a therapeutic level, a common and agreed-on definition of the problem must be composed. This can be a challenge as oftentimes people perceive problems quite differently because clinical problems are usually complex and multifaceted. Providers see problems from their perspective or "facet" of the problem and can perceive that to be in conflict with the other professions, but in actuality, each view is one facet of the major problem, and the fact that each view is represented is the beauty of interprofessional work. For example, the nurse may see a patient's low health literacy in understanding the importance of taking their heart failure medications as the main problem, while a social worker may see a patient's restrictive insurance coverage and lack of private pay financial resources to pay for medications as the main problem, and the physician may see the hemodynamic instability of the patient as the main problem. However, these issues are all contributory to a shared problem of controlling heart failure and using each member's skill set to work collaboratively to address each facet of the situation (Bojeun, 2013).

Helping team members take a moment to briefly step back or "zoom out" and look at the problem from a bird's-eye view is critical to ensuring the group maintains a cohesive mission and vision with shared goals. Depicting problems on a common area whiteboard where interprofessional meetings take place and where it can be kept visible during future interactions to remind the group of the collaborative purpose is a great way to visualize this for the team and keep the common shared vision at the forefront. Cause-and-effect diagrams or fishbone diagrams (see Figure 5.1) are a great way to accomplish this (Institute for Healthcare Improvement, 2023).

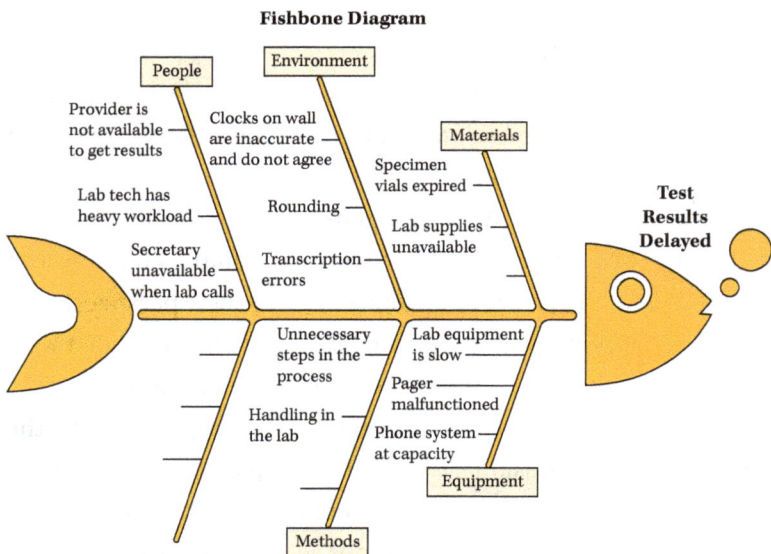

Fishbone Diagram

People

Environment

Provider is not available to get results

Clocks on wall are inaccurate and do not agree

Materials

Lab tech has heavy workload

Rounding

Specimen vials expired

Test Results Delayed

Secretary unavailable when lab calls

Transcription errors

Lab supplies unavailable

Unnecessary steps in the process

Lab equipment is slow

Handling in the lab

Pager malfunctioned

Phone system at capacity

Equipment

Methods

FIGURE 5.1   Example cause-and-effect (fishbone) diagram.

ELABORATIVE BEHAVIOR

Tempering professional identifications while increasing collaborative goal setting usually results in increases in elaborative behavior. Elaborative team behavior is the open exchange of information and ideas while seeking clarification on differing perspectives. There is an immense amount of knowledge and skill sets in an interprofessional team, so this is crucial formulating a plan consensus. A spirit of trust and openness is key, in which team members feel comfortable asking questions. Elaborative communication styles help the team collaborate to meet the shared goals (Salas et al., 2017).

Advanced-Level Sub-Competency 9.3j: Leadership Skills in Professional Activities and Organizations

SCENARIO 3

Mrs. Jones is a 70-year-old female with a medical history of hypertension, osteoarthritis, Crohn's disease, and total knee replacement 5 years ago. She is at her primary care provider's annual physical with Gary Smith, APRN. During the medication reconciliation with the office's MA, Mrs. Jones shares that tomorrow she will be starting amoxicillin in preparation to have her teeth cleaned at her dentist office. During the visit, Gary asks Mrs. Jones why she is being prescribed the antibiotic and learns that her dentist always prescribes this before every cleaning because of her knee replacement history and concerns for joint infection from oral bacteria entering the patient's bloodstream during the cleaning. Gary knows that this used to be a common practice; however, the clinical practice guidelines published by the American Dental Association and American Academy of Orthopedic Surgeons in 2010 recommend against prescribing prophylactic antibiotics for patients who have had joint replacements because of no causal association and the high risk of antibiotic resistance issues, in particular, *Clostridium difficile (C. diff)*–associated gastroenteritis. He also knows that Mrs. Smith is even at a higher risk for *C. diff* than the general population because of her age and gastrointestinal condition. Gary tells Mrs. Smith, "Do not take that antibiotic; that is an outdated practice." Mrs. Smith calls the office 5 days later, very upset. She says that when she showed up to her appointment to have her teeth cleaned and when she told the dentist that she did not take the antibiotic, they canceled her appointment and would not clean her teeth.

Discussion Questions

1. It may seem that the two providers have different goals that are in conflict. However, what shared mission are they on? How could highlighting the shared vision help this situation?
2. How could Gary make this more of an collaborative experience between the two professions?
3. When thinking about this scenario, do you think the dentist and Gary could consider Mrs. Smith as part of the team and elaborate on communications with her as well? How can considering patients as part of the team help? What problems can arise?

"Every well-prepared, successful nurse is a leader" (AACN, 2023, para. 1). Specifically, APRNs should make an effort to serve in leadership roles on organizational committees and be active in health policy with diverse groups of professions. Examples include QA/QI committees, ethics boards, and legislative action groups at the state and national level. Maintaining a collaborative character with other professions while holding them accountable to nursing values can be a challenge. Advocating for individual patients in specific scenarios often comes instinctively to nurses. However, advanced levels of advocacy, including with policy and legislation, is exponentially important. Analysis of system-level effects of patient care, particularly cost, are hot topics at the professional and administrative levels. Many nurses don't like to talk about money and politics, but don't be intimidated by the boardroom; society wants and needs you there! According to a survey conducted by *The New York Times*, the Commonwealth Fund, and the Harvard T.H. Chan School of Public Health in 2019, Americans trust nurses the most to improve the U.S. health care system; 58% of respondents gave nurses the vote of confidence, which was the only profession to receive majority support. Just under a third of respondents trusted physicians, and even fewer trusted hospitals (18%) or the federal government (6%). A main reason is because successful nursing leaders always strive to pair critical thinking skills with our core values (human dignity, integrity, autonomy, altruism, and social justice) to motivate change. This is often referred to as the "nursing lens" (Patton et al., 2014).

An important way our lens is valuable in interprofessional teams is our focus on addressing health disparities. Disenfranchised groups rely on the compassion and humanity of nurses to advocate for their needs at all levels. The advanced-level nurse must be skilled in detecting if the moral compass of an organization strays off course from ensuring health equity and exercising moral courage when necessary to influence other professions to support the health of all individuals of all social backgrounds and circumstances. Cost-effective care can and should be ethically competent care, although it may require innovative approaches.

Demonstrating leadership skills is different than being *the* leader. Misconceptions about leadership include the belief that it means being in charge or making all of the decisions. Rather, a participatory approach is a more powerful form of leadership, with judicious use of assertiveness. This calls for involving informed and influential stakeholders in understanding the complex interdependencies of a system to support change. See Chapter 2 for a more detailed look at different leadership styles.

Advanced-Level Sub-Competency 6.2j: Foster Positive Team Dynamics to Strengthen Desired Outcomes

SCENARIO 4

Judy is a primary care provider APRN who has worked at an outpatient internal medicine clinic owned by a large health system for 15 years, and she specializes in geriatric care for a low-income population. She is serving on an outpatient quality improvement committee in her health system. The committee consists of one nurse (Judy), three hospital executives, one pharmacist, and one physician. The group focuses on evaluating clinical procedures to streamline processes and evaluate clinical practice guidelines to ensure up-to-date and cost-effective care. It has been highlighted that the clinic's medical assistants spend an exorbitant amount of time calling patients to notify them about their test results. Most patients have a low level of health literacy, so they often have questions about their results. This is causing other work to be tardy because of the time the MAs are spending on the phone. Most of the committee members agree on instituting a new policy that patients will be notified of their results through a smartphone app only (no more live phone calls), and if they have a question about their results they must make an appointment to come and see their provider to discuss their questions. Judy knows that most of her patient panel has difficulty using the health system's mobile app, if they even have a smartphone at all. Additionally, many have mobility and transportation challenges, so to require them to make an appointment to come to the office will be a barrier to them to be able to receive timely knowledge about their health status. She feels that this new policy will disenfranchise her patient population, whose social determinants of health do not support using mobile apps and getting to appointments.

Key points for advocating for health equity in the interdisciplinary team (Patton et al., 2014) include the following:

- Luckily, Judy's past 15 years of practice at the organization has given her time to build a positive rapport with other clinicians. She always seeks opportunities to collaborate with all professions. This is key to being an influential leader on an interdisciplinary team. Build bridges, don't burn them, during your career.

- Stories are almost always more influential than debating alone, and all nurses have stories. Judy shares a scenario in which a patient's COVID test is positive but the patient does not get the message in a timely manner because they don't have their smartphone notifications on their phone set up. She illustrates the potential public health ramifications and spread of disease in this scenario.
- Participatory approach: Judy can invite speakers from her clinic who she knows have shared similar experiences to the QI meeting.
- Compromise/collaboration: She could suggest a tiered approach to result notification instead of an "all-or-nothing" approach. For example, results indicative of infections receive phone calls, whereas others such as negative preventative screening results can use the smartphone app.
- Innovation: Judy makes a point to be savvy and up-to-date on billing and coding practices for her practice. She is aware of opportunities to be reimbursed for time spent on the phone with patients. She asks to form a small committee (participatory approach) to create a coding manual for the clinics and training for office staff to capture the ways the clinics can seek reimbursement for the phone calls, such as through chronic care management billing and telemedicine codes.

CONCLUSION

The primary responsibility of health care providers at all levels is to promote positive patient outcomes. In order for patient care to be at its best, all of the members of a health care team need to perform optimally. Clear communication of the roles of members of the team is vitally important. The nurse needs to be able to articulate their role on the team. If the nurse is the leader, they should be responsive to the rest of the team. All members of a health care team are needed to facilitate quality care. The roles and responsibilities of each collaborating member should be clear to the entire team. If conflict arises, the team members should work together to manage the conflict and communicate effectively.

KEY POINTS

- Understanding the roles and responsibilities of the nurse and other members of a team is a critical foundation on which to build workflows and promote success.
- Team dynamics can be functional or dysfunctional, and nurses have an important responsibility to ensure all roles support successful patient care.
- It is important for nurses to lead efforts to engage many disciplines, within their workplace and beyond, to facilitate quality improvement and policy change that supports patients.

ACTIVITIES

Activity 1: Introducing the Concept of Team Dynamics

Think about the times you have worked on teams and answer the following questions:

- Is there a time when you felt that the team was functional? Is there a time when you felt the team was dysfunctional?
- Can you put into words the way that you felt in each situation?
- Did the team's understanding of each other's roles and responsibilities impact the team's function? How?

Activity 2: Shared Goals for Patient Care

Work with another student and make a cause-and-effect (fishbone) diagram, related to a common concern such as patient falls or medication errors. A template is available through the Institute of Healthcare Improvement (2023). Identify, on the diagram, which professions might be responsible for each item listed.

Activity 3: Professional Diversity and Identities

Look up the professional organization of a profession that you may not know well and answer the following questions:

- What is the profession's educational requirements?
- What is the pathway to licensing and/or certification? For example, are internships required? How often do they recertify? Are continuing education hours required?
- Are there any current initiatives, such as policy change, that the profession is currently pursuing?
- Identify one thing you learned that you did not know before about this profession.
- Was there anything that you were surprised to find? Do you feel more or less connected or comfortable with the profession's background? The next time you meet someone from that profession at a party, what will you ask them?

REFERENCES

American Association of Colleges of Nursing. (2021). *The essentials: Core competencies for professional nursing education.* https://www.aacnnursing.org/Essentials

American Association of Colleges of Nursing. (2023). *Leadership.* https://www.aacnnursing.org/5B-Tool-Kit/Themes/Leadership

Americans' values and beliefs about national health insurance reform. (2019). *Medical Benefits, 36*(12), 5–6.

Bojeun, M. C. (2013). *Program management leadership: Creating successful team dynamics.* CRC Press.

Cruess, R. L., Cruess, S. R., Boudreau, J. D., Snell, L., & Steinert, Y. (2014). Reframing medical education to support professional identity formation. *Academic Medicine: Journal of the Association of American Medical Colleges, 89*(11), 1446–1451. https://doi.org/10.1097/ACM.0000000000000427

Dajani, D. & Uddin, L. (2015). Demystifying cognitive flexibility: Implications for clinical and developmental neuroscience. *Trends in Neurosciences, 38*(9) 571–578.

Fitzgerald, J. A., & Teal, G. (2004). Health reform, professional identity and occupational sub-cultures: The changing interprofessional relations between doctors and nurses. *Contemporary Nurse, 16*(1–2), 9–19.

Institute for Healthcare Improvement. (2023). *Tools: Cause and effect diagram.* https://www.ihi.org/resources/Pages/Tools/CauseandEffectDiagram.aspx

Interprofessional Education Collaborative Expert Panel. (2011). *Core competencies for interprofessional collaborative practice: Report of an expert panel.* Interprofessional Education Collaborative.

Interprofessional Education Collaborative. (2016). *Core competencies for interprofessional collaborative practice: 2016 update. Interprofessional Education Collaborative.*

Koch, I., Poljac, E., Muller, H., & Kiesel, A. (2018). Cognitive structure, flexibilityand plasticity in human multitasking: An intergrative review of dial-task and task-switching research, *Psychological Bulletin, 144*(6) 557–583.

Lingard, L., Reznick, R., DeVito, I., & Espin, S. (2002). Forming professional identities on the health care team: Discursive constructions of the "other" in the operating room. *Medical Education, 36*(8), 728–734.

Mitchell, R., Parker, V., Giles, M., & Boyle, B. (2014). The ABC of health care team dynamics: Understanding complex affective, behavioral, and cognitive dynamics in interprofessional teams. *Health Care Manage Rev., 39*(1), 1–9. https://doi.org/10.1097/HCM.0b013e3182766504

Patton, R. M., Zalon, M. L., & Ludwick, R. (2014). *Nurses making policy: From bedside to boardroom.* Springer.

Salas, E., Vessey, W. B., & Landon, L. B. (2017). *Team dynamics over time.* Emerald.

St Martin, L., Harripaul, A, Antonacci, R., Laframboise, D., Purden, M (2015) Advanced beginner to competent practitioner: New graduate nurses' perception of strategies that facilitate or hinder development, *Clinical Education of Nurses, 46*(9) 392–400.

CREDIT

CHAPTER 6

Respect

Janna Draine Kinney, DNP, RN, CCRN, and Me'Chelle Hayes, MSN, RN, FNP-BC

KEY AACN COMPETENCIES, SUB-COMPETENCIES, AND CONCEPTS

Domain 5: Quality and Safety

Competency 5.3 Contribute to a culture of provider and work environment safety.

- ***Entry-Level Sub-Competency 5.3d*** Recognize one's role in sustaining a just culture reflecting civility and respect.
- ***Advanced-Level Sub-Competency 5.3f*** Foster a just culture reflecting civility and respect.

Domain 6: Interprofessional Partnerships

Competency 6.1 Communicate in a manner that facilitates a partnership approach to quality care delivery.

- ***Advanced Level Sub-Competency 6.1i*** Role-model respect for diversity, equity, and inclusion in team-based communications.

Competency 6.4 Work with other professions to maintain a climate of mutual learning, respect and shared values.

Continued

Continued

- ***Entry-Level Sub-Competency 6.4a*** Demonstrate an awareness of one's biases and how they may affect mutual respect and communication with team members.

- ***Entry-Level Sub-Competency 6.4b*** Demonstrate respect for the perspectives and experiences of other professions.

- ***Advanced-Level Sub-Competency 6.4g*** Integrate diversity, equity, and inclusion into team practices.

Domain 9: Professionalism

Competency 9.3 Demonstrate accountability to the individual, society, and the profession.

- ***Entry-Level Sub-Competency 9.3f*** Demonstrate adherence to a culture of civility.

Concepts for Nursing Practice

- Communication
- Diversity, equity, and inclusion
- Ethics

KEY TERMS

Respect	Incivility
Implicit bias	Microaggression
Civility	Integrity
Bullying	

INTRODUCTION: WHAT IS RESPECT?

Respect is a concept central to most health care professions and professionalism in general (Persily, 2013). For many providers, respect is included in their respective codes of ethics (American Medical Association [AMA], 2016; American Nurses Association [ANA], 2015). *Respect* is a positive feeling or action shown toward someone or something considered essential or held in high esteem or regard (Merriam-Webster, 2022). It is also the process of honoring someone by exhibiting care, concern, or consideration for their needs or feelings regardless of how you feel about them (Healey, 2012; Merriam-Webster, 2022). Respect in nursing recognizes and appreciates each patient's inherent dignity, worth, and unique attributes (ANA, 2021). It involves treating patients with kindness, compassion, understanding, and consideration for their feelings, needs, and preferences (ANA, 2021).

In addition to showing respect for patients, health care providers should also demonstrate respect for their colleagues, supervisors, and other interprofessional team members. Respect is valued in interprofessional collaboration; is intrinsic to a positive, collaborative relationship; and is an important component of achieving patient-centered care (Sokol-Hessner et al., 2018). This includes working collaboratively, communicating effectively, and valuing the contributions of others. Conducting oneself with integrity is another facet of respect. A person who behaves consistently with *integrity* acts in accordance with their personal moral values and upholds ethical standards (Holsinger & Carlton, 2018; Persily, 2013). When working in an interprofessional team, members must prioritize communication as well as the needs of the stakeholders over their own (Holsinger & Carlton, 2018). To foster respect in the interprofessional setting, all team members and the work of the team should be treated with respect despite any friction that may arise between individuals on the team (Persily, 2013).

Disrespect and Incivility

The inverse of respectful behaviors (or *civility*) is frequently called incivility rather than disrespect. Workplace incivility is a social interaction that consists of "low intensity deviant behavior ... in violation of workplace norms for mutual respect" (Andersson & Pearson, 1999, p. 457). Uncivil behaviors are rude and discourteous and display a lack of respect for others (Andersson & Pearson, 1999) They are also 10 times more likely to occur in health care settings than acts of physical violence and aggression (Hutton & Gates, 2008). Ciocco (2018, p. 18) acknowledges that incivility can occur as a response to a stressful work environment, particularly when health care professionals are navigating the multitude of expectations and demands of their profession.

Uncivil and disrespectful behaviors are typically distinguished by their passivity. Some examples of these behaviors include, but are not limited to, belittling comments and gestures (eye rolling, lip sounds, sighs, groans, and mutters), skipping greetings, sarcasm, social exclusion, gossiping, silent treatment, and cellular phone usage while having interactions with others (Bar-David, 2018). Nonpassive behaviors can include gossiping, name calling, spreading rumors, public criticism, refusing to assist a coworker (ANA, 2015), or failing to act when warranted when other coworkers are being treated disrespectfully (Clark, 2017).

SCENARIO 1

During interprofessional rounds on a medical intensive care unit (MICU), Susan, a veteran MICU nurse, discusses overnight events and the plan of care for a critically ill patient on the unit. Jaylen, a new physician assistant caring for the patient and entering orders, asks Susan to clarify the information she has provided the team. Susan rolls her eyes, does not provide the requested information, and continues to discuss the patient with other interprofessional team members. This illustrates a situation in which one interprofessional team member displayed uncivil behaviors toward another.

Discussion Questions

1. What behaviors were uncivil or disrespectful?
2. How can these behaviors impact patient safety and outcomes?
3. How can these behaviors impact other members of the interprofessional team?

In scenario 1, Susan rolls her eyes, does not provide the required information to the requesting team member, and excludes Jaylen from the remainder of interprofessional rounds. Though these behaviors are low intensity and seemingly harmless, they can lead to further disrespectful and uncivil behaviors and interfere with communication within the team. Disrespectful and uncivil behaviors among health care team members can negatively affect individuals, team members, and patient safety and outcomes (Clarke, 2019). These behaviors affect not only the person being targeted but also bystanders, stakeholders, and organizations. In instances when incivility remains unaddressed, these situations can become safety concerns and financially impact the organization (Clark, 2017). Some of the more tangible outcomes include decreased work effort, time at work, quality of work, and decreased commitment to the organization (Porath & Pearson, 2013). Those who have been on the receiving end of incivility also report losing work time worrying about the incident and ultimately leaving the organization due to the behaviors (Porath & Pearson, 2013). Incivility in the workplace also negatively affects those who witness it. Houshmand et al. (2012) found that even indirect incivility leads to higher turnover intentions. These consequences also occur in the health care setting, as seen in Table 6.1.

It is worth noting that incivility and disrespectful behaviors are not synonymous with microaggression or bullying, which typically result from incivility and a lack of respect.

Microaggressions

Microaggressions are intentional or unintentional behaviors that express hostile, derogatory, or negative attitudes toward marginalized groups (Ehie et al., 2021). Microaggressions typically communicate some sort of bias toward a marginalized group (Limbong, 2020). Another definition is the "everyday verbal, non-verbal, and environmental slights, snubs, or insults, intentional or

TABLE 6.1   **Work-Related Outcomes of Interprofessional Incivility**

Patient safety and outcomes	• Bullying and incivility lead to decreased levels of communication, teamwork, and collaboration, which are the underpinnings of effective interprofessional patient care (Adams & Maykut, 2015). • When tension is elevated, and incivility is present in-patient care areas, staff cannot perform at their best, resulting in poor patient care (Martin & Zadinsky, 2022; Woelfle & McCaffrey, 2007).
Stress-related health problems	• Incivility from managers or coworkers has been linked to anxiety among new graduate nurses (Martin & Zadinsky, 2022). • Incivility from sources in the emergency department can lead to decreased levels of psychological safety for physicians (Martin & Zadinsky, 2022). • Incivility from coworkers and supervisors is linked to increased levels of fatigue and burnout (Martin & Zadinsky, 2022). • Nurses experiencing bullying display lower levels of self-esteem. self-hatred, and depression (Adams & Maykut, 2015; ANA, 2015).
Intention to leave one's job	• When workers are bullied at work, they have a stronger inclination to leave the workplace where the bullying is present (Clark, 2017; Houshmand et al., 2012). • Working in a unit with a considerable amount of bullying is linked to higher employee turnover intentions (Clark, 2017; Houshmand et al., 2012).
Increased financial cost	• Incivility-related production losses amount to nearly $300,000 (Hutton & Gates, 2008). • Training and retention of health care providers, no matter the role, has led to increased costs for hospital systems (Houshmand et al., 2012; Martin & Zadinsky, 2022). • Across 17 industries, workers who have experienced incivility have decreased their work quality or time spent at work (Porath & Pearson, 2013). • Incivility and disrespect can push patients and health care workers away from hospital systems, leading to increased turnover costs and loss of revenue (Sokol-Hessner et al., 2018).

unintentional, that communicate hostile, derogatory, or negative messages to target persons based solely on their marginalized group membership" (Garibay, 2014, p. 10, Sue et al., 2007). Typically, microaggressions are related to race or ethnicity. However, in the interprofessional setting, the term can refer to behaviors or comments expressed toward other health care professionals who are often dismissed, marginalized, or underappreciated in the health care setting.

Microaggressions can be further defined as three different types: microassaults, microinsults, or microinvalidation. Microassaults are explicitly derogatory and are meant to hurt the intended victim with name-calling, avoidant behavior, or purposefully discriminatory actions or words (Sue et al., 2007). Microassaults are typically conscious and deliberate but are expressed privately (Sue et al., 2007). For this discussion, microassaults, though classified as a type of microaggression, will be further discussed as a bullying behavior as it is intentional.

Microinsults are characterized by verbal communication in which the perpetrator conveys rudeness and insensitivity to the victim (Sue et al., 2007). These snubs are unknown to the perpetrator but are acutely felt by the victim, for example, asking a younger-looking colleague about their qualifications or credentials. Microinsults can also be nonverbal, such as when a White colleague fails to make eye contact with a Black colleague or when an attending physician does not recognize the contributions of other team members during interprofessional rounds.

Microinvalidations occur when other health care team members invalidate another person's experiences. In practice, this may look like a member of the health care team describing a racist or sexist encounter and being told that they misunderstood what was said or that their perception of the situation was inaccurate. Microinvalidations dismiss the victim's lived experiences, thoughts, or feelings (Parikh & Leschied, 2022). See Table 6.2

for examples of microaggressions, microassaults, microinsults, and microinvalidations.

TABLE 6.2 **Examples of Microaggressions, Microassaults, Microinsults, and Microinvalidations**

Microaggression	A provider neglects to ask about a patient's family history because "*those people usually do not know who their father is.*"
Microassault	Members of the interprofessional team frequently refer to a nurse as "Skippy" because the nurse sometimes stutters when she speaks.
Microinsult	Two providers are meeting for the first time. One provider says to the other, "Your name is so exotic; you must not be from here. Where are you from?"
Microinvalidation	While recounting an interaction with a patient and the patient referred to the provider using a racial epithet, the provider was told, "I am sure they meant no harm; they are from a different generation. It is not a big deal."

SCENARIO 2

A hospital unit hosts an educational simulation and learning activity for interprofessional learners. The learners in the group represent a variety of health care roles and professions with varying levels of experience. During the activity, the session facilitators repeatedly refer to the physician learners by their professional "doctor" title. This continues throughout the simulation, while the other learners in the group are addressed by first name only. During the debriefing session for the simulation, the facilitator continues to refer to the physician learners using their professional titles and the other learners by their first names. The physician learners refer to one another as "colleagues" and to the other learners as "the nurses" or "the physical therapists," never referring to them as colleagues.

Discussion Questions

1. Do the actions of the physician learners and facilitators qualify as microaggressions? If so, how?
2. How do the choices in language for members of the interprofessional team impact team morale?
3. How might the way participants refer to each other such as using professional titles or "colleagues" impact collaboration?
4. How could the learners improve their word choices and improve the culture of the interprofessional team to show respect in their communication with one another?
5. Consider that you are an advanced practice provider on this interprofessional team. When introducing the team to patients and families, the physicians refer to each other by their professional titles and other team members. How would this impact collaboration? How would this impact the patient's relationship with the team?

Avoiding language and behaviors that include microaggressions is essential to fostering respect in the interprofessional setting. Several strategies to avoid microaggressions while communicating with interprofessional collaborators include acknowledging the power of language and behaviors, understanding that microaggressions can transcend race and ethnicity, and validating the victim's perspective of the microaggression (Holtschneider & Park, 2021). These, and other strategies, are further discussed in Table 6.3.

Bullying

As previously noted, bullying and incivility are not synonymous. Incivility may or may not have negative intent and is not considered a form of violence. *Bullying* is "repeated, unwanted, harmful actions intended to humiliate, offend, and cause distress in the recipient" (ANA, n.d, para. 2). Additionally, bullying is used to control the recipient (Ciocco, 2018, p. 19). Bullying can be described in several ways: workplace bullying, horizontal violence, and lateral violence.

Workplace bullying is marked by threatening and humiliating behaviors intended to sabotage another's work or egregious verbal abuse (The Joint Commission, 2021). These behaviors are often a reflection of the perceived hierarchical stratifications that exist in health care settings. For example, when physicians or advanced practice providers bully those perceived as "lesser than" such as nurses, nurses bully certified nursing assistants, or health professionals bully environmental service workers (Fink-Samnick, 2015). When there is an imbalance of power within the interprofessional team, the team's effectiveness will be impacted (Okpala, 2021).

In contrast, lateral and horizontal violence happens when people are both victims of a situation of dominance and turn on one another rather than opposing the power structure or perpetrator who oppressed them both (Fink-Samnick, 2015). McLean et al. (2023) define *power* as the ability to control, direct, and influence others, including prevalent norms and practices embedded within institutional structures and systems of society that favor some groups over others. A power structure refers to systems used to control others. When power is used to exert burdensome restraints over others, it is deemed as oppression. With the increasing demands from health care systems placed on interprofessional team members, frustrations can quickly arise, and colleagues can become easy targets for previously internalized emotions. In some instances, bullying in health care occurs and is permitted due to the perceived hierarchy of health care professionals. Because of the effects of perceived hierarchy and power held by interprofessional team members, the health care field has some of the highest rates of bullying and lateral violence in the workplace (Fink-Samnick, 2015).

Bullying and lateral violence are detrimental to the interprofessional team. A highly functional team emphasizes collaboration, cooperation, and respect to deliver patient-centered care. When bullying and violence are present, team member cohesion is negatively impacted. The Interprofessional Education Collaborative (IPEC, 2021) asserts that bullying and violence are detrimental to one of its core competencies: working with individuals of other professions to maintain a climate of mutual respect.

APPLICATION TO PRACTICE: HOW DO WE FOSTER INTERPROFESSIONAL RESPECT?

Being treated with respect is crucial to working in an interprofessional team and impacts patient care, health care worker safety, and the workplace environment. Being respectful is more than just being nice, complimentary, or kind. It involves creating and utilizing strategies that cultivate respect, prevent microaggressions and bullying, and provide frameworks for reporting and resolving incidents related to disrespect and incivility.

Strategies to Cultivate Respect

Nurses can take leadership roles in cultivating respect in health care teams through intentional planning and engagement with team members and patients. The following section outlines strategies that nurses and other health care professionals (HCP) can use to create a more respective working environment in health care.

RAISING AWARENESS OF THE BENEFITS OF RESPECT

One of the first strategies to cultivate respectful interprofessional teams is raising awareness of respect and its benefits. Uncivil behaviors are often unconscious and respectful behaviors are intentional. Acknowledging, appreciating, and valuing the diversity of the interprofessional team can facilitate respectful working conditions (Healey, 2012). Helping team members recognize the importance of their conscious and unconscious behaviors, their impact on other team members, and their impact on outcomes is crucial to ensuring a respectful working environment and relationship. This can be accomplished with messaging, positive reinforcement of respectful behavior by team members, and providing education about the importance of respectful behaviors, incivility's consequences, and the repercussions of both behaviors on team members and patient outcomes.

EXAMINING IMPLICIT BIAS

Implicit bias is the automatic or implicit processes of judgments and social behaviors. It refers to the attitudes and stereotypes that unconsciously affect understanding, actions, and decisions (Kirwan Institute for the Study of Race and Ethnicity, 2015). The phenomenon encompasses favorable and unfavorable assessments that are generally involuntary and occur unconsciously but can manifest in decision-making, nonverbal behaviors, and interactions with categories of people, which are all important when working in an interprofessional team (Fitzgerald & Hurst, 2017). Implicit association test results have indicated that health care professionals may hold biases in many areas related to patient care. Higher levels of bias can negatively impact surgical outcomes; increase the length of hospital stays; and affect patient–provider interactions, provider–provider interactions, treatment adherence for patients, and patient health outcomes (Hall et al., 2015; Kirwan Institute for the Study of Race and Ethnicity, 2015). If patients are aware of provider biases or feel discriminated against, they may choose not to participate in health care screenings or visits, delay seeking help and filling prescriptions, and score the quality of the care received lower (Hall et al., 2015). Examining and understanding one's biases is crucial in cultivating respect with patients and other interprofessional team members.

BUILD TEAM SUPPORT AND BUY-IN

Raising awareness of the importance of workplace civility and respect can promote individual buy-in. If team members feel a personal responsibility to ensure respect dominates their interactions, the team will work more effectively and productively and have better outcomes. However, individual buy-in is not enough; developing and supporting people, systems, and practices that promote respect and civility is also critical. Creating and supporting systems, people, and practices that promote respect and civility ensures that those actively participating in creating a respectful team environment will remain engaged in respectful practices and will encourage those who are not active participants (Sokol-Hessner et al., 2018).

PROMOTE ACCOUNTABILITY

Creating civil and respectful teamwork environments is the goal, but incivility is likely to occur when working with professionals and patients from various backgrounds and belief systems. Finding ways to promote accountability when these incidents occur is critical to preventing harm to team members and patients and averting further incidences of incivility and bullying.

PARTNER WITH PATIENTS AND FAMILIES

Health care professionals are not the only victims of disrespect. For patients and families, disrespect and incivility have been associated with a worse experience, a lower likelihood of perceiving care as quality, and a lower likelihood of seeking care in the same facility (Sokol-Hessner et al., 2018). Partnering with patients and families and treating them as members of the interprofessional team can alleviate these concerns. Tactics to address each of these strategies are discussed in Table 6.3.

TABLE 6.3 **Specific Tactics to Cultivate Respect in Interprofessional Teams**

Strategies	Specific Tactics by AACN Defined by Nursing Education Level
Raise awareness	Entry level • Participate in respect and incivility training (Sokol-Hessner et al., 2018).
	Advanced level • Provide educational resources (written materials, classes/in-services, bulletin boards, etc.) regarding the importance of respect and civility to all members of the interprofessional team. • Share data about the benefits of respect and the consequences of incivility (Sokol-Hessner et al., 2018).
Examine implicit bias	Entry level • Take a self-administered implicit association test (IAT) to determine areas of bias (Project Implicit, 2011). • Work to mitigate bias, more information available from The Ohio State University (n.d.). • Consider implicit biases when caring for patients and families.
	Advanced level • Take a self-administered implicit association test (IAT) to determine area(s) of bias (Project Implicit, 2011). • Work to mitigate bias (The Ohio State University, n.d.). • Consider implicit biases when establishing a holistic plan of care for patients and families. • Lead organizational and systems-level change to address implicit bias in health care.
Build team support	Entry level • Allow team members to define what constitutes respect in their respective settings (Sokol-Hessner, et al., 2018) and on their teams. • Allow team members to provide stories and examples of respect or disrespect; this will provide concrete examples of acceptable and unacceptable behaviors.
	Advanced level • Facilitate the opportunity for teams to complete a team assessment of skills and beliefs. • Encourage team members to set group norms or a group contract for respectful behaviors (Linabary & Castro, 2021).
Develop and support people, systems, and practices that promote respect and civility	Entry level • Share stories of respect and the impact on the team or patient outcomes (Sokol-Hessner et al., 2018). • Use public communication (social media, intra-organization newsletter) to highlight respectful colleagues and their impact. • Use public communication to reiterate the importance of respect and civility (Sokol-Hessner et al., 2018).
	Advanced level • Develop or support recognition programs to acknowledge and commend team members who embody respect and respectful practices (Sokol-Hessner et al., 2018). • Conduct "respect rounds" and collect examples of respect to be celebrated (Sokol-Hessner et al., 2018). • Consider the impact of team decision-making on creating and maintaining respectful environments (Sokol-Hessner et al., 2018).

Strategies	Specific Tactics by AACN Defined by Nursing Education Level
Promote accountability	**Entry level** • Conduct team and self–check-ins to account for adherence to group norms/beliefs and respectful behaviors. • Use systems to report incidents of incivility or bullying. • Debrief after incidents to make meaningful and timely improvements (Sokol-Hessner et al., 2018).
	Advanced level • Develop systems to report incidents of incivility or bullying. • Develop policies and procedures that address incidences of disrespect/incivility/bullying (Sokol-Hessner et al., 2018). • Continually evaluate systems and teamwork to ensure respect is present. • Ensure that disrespect is addressed in a timely fashion with all parties involved (Sokol-Hessner et al., 2018).
Partner with patients and families	**Entry level** • Emphasize that patient-centered care is an equally important domain of quality in the team and organization (Sokol-Hessner et al., 2018). • Use culturally appropriate care. • Continually consider language and cultural barriers to care. • Use empathy when caring for patients and families. • Utilize patient and family engagement programs (Sokol-Hessner et al., 2018). • Incorporate patient and family goals into team goals and outcomes when possible.
	Advanced level • Partner with community organizations that advocate for populations experiencing health care disparities (Sokol-Hessner et al., 2018). • Develop patient and family engagement programs (Sokol-Hessner et al., 2018). • Develop methods to communicate standards of respect with patients and family members effectively (Sokol-Hessner et al., 2018).

Strategies to Prevent and Address Microaggressions and Bullying

Microaggressions and bullying differ from incivility. Uncivil behaviors may or may not have a harmful intent, while microaggressions are "brief and commonplace verbal, behavioral, and environmental indignities … that communicate hostile, derogatory, or negative slights and insults that potentially have harmful or unpleasant psychological impact on the target person or group" (Sue et al., 2007, p. 271). Microaggressions can also be intentional or unintentional but typically are leveraged toward a marginalized group. Strategies to prevent and address microaggressions and bullying on an interpersonal level are described in detail in Table 6.4.

TABLE 6.4 **Specific Tactics to Address and Prevent Microaggressions and Bullying**

Strategies	Specific Tactics
Acknowledge the behavior	• If the incident occurs within a team setting, provide examples of microaggressions and bullying using brief case studies or videos. After discussing the educational material, provide scenarios and ask team members to identify the behavior presented (Heath et al., 2021; Parikh & Leschied, 2022). • If the behavior occurs between individuals, clearly express your disagreement with the statement to the speaker—with phrases such as "I do not agree with what you said" or "I do not support the actions that took place" (Parikh & Leschied, 2022).
Inquire	• Ask the speaker to elaborate on their statement to understand their perspective better. Avoid using "why" questions to decrease defensiveness and instead use phrases such as "What makes you ask that?" or "What makes you believe that?" (Kenney, 2014).
Paraphrase and reflect	• Paraphrasing can decrease defensiveness and show that the listener is seeking understanding. Phrases such as "You're saying …" and "It sounds like you're saying …" can be helpful when paraphrasing (Kenney, 2014).
Reframe the belief	• Reframing the belief or statement allows the speaker to uncover their bias or mis-held belief. Phrases such as "What would happen if another colleague said this to you?" or "What would happen if …" can be helpful when reframing (Kenney, 2014).

Strategies	Specific Tactics
Using impact, "I," and preference statements	• Impact and "I" statements are clear and nonthreatening ways to address an issue directly; for example, "I felt upset/disappointed/disrespected when you said/did ..." • Preference statements clearly address one's needs and preferences so there is no room for ambiguity. For example, "It would be helpful to me/our patient(s) if ..." or "I would like it if you used my correct pronouns" (Kenney, 2014).
Revisit the situation	• Unaddressed microaggressions and instances of bullying can be just as harmful as the actual event (Kenney, 2014). • Taking a time-out and revisiting the situation can provide a level of privacy for the parties involved in a low-stakes environment.

On a systemic level, teams and organizations should address areas in which instances of bullying and microaggressions can be eradicated or prevented. This can be completed by carrying out team and organizational assessments to inform and create prevention programs, creating policies and resources that address recourse for instances of bullying and uncivil behavior, and providing ongoing education for conflict management (AORN Staff, 2021).

SCENARIO 3

Benjamin is a respiratory therapist working at a hospital and sees patients on many different units. Benjamin finishes the change of shift report and goes to the medical telemetry unit to see a patient. Benjamin steps into the hallway after administering medication to the patient. As he turns the corner, he hears a cry for help from the patient's room. He rushes back into the room to see the patient lying on the ground after a fall. After assessing the patient, he calls the physical therapist, walking past the room, for help. After getting the patient back to bed and leaves the room, the physical therapist turns to Benjamin and berates him, calling him incompetent for allowing the patient to fall.

Discussion Questions

1. Which of the strategies in Table 6.4 would be most effective at fostering and creating respect in this situation? Why?
2. Are there any strategies listed that may not be helpful in this scenario? Why or why not?
3. Benjamin chooses not to address the physical therapist's remarks in the moment, but he frequently works with him. How can Benjamin revisit the situation during a future encounter to ensure a respectful working relationship?

CONCLUSION

Creating a respectful and civil environment for patients and coworkers is the responsibility of all HCPs. Nurses can address these issues within their interprofessional team and within their organization in formal and informal leadership roles. While the issues around respect and civility are complex and it may feel daunting to address them, there are concrete steps nurses and other HCPs can take to build a more supportive and welcoming health care system. First, it is important to understand how attitudes, biases, and behaviors can contribute to incivility and impact patients and HCPs. Incivility, such as microaggressions and bullying, harms working relationships, contributes to low-quality patient care, and increases stress, staff turnover, and health care costs. Second, taking time for self-reflection and examining personal implicit biases helps individuals become more self-aware and better able to mitigate their own biases. Third, nurses and other HCPs can foster interprofessional respect by raising awareness, building team support and buy-in, promoting accountability, and partnering with patients and families. Finally, learning specific approaches to address and prevent microaggressions and bullying helps to create a culture in which those behaviors are not tolerated and all members of the interprofessional team are respected.

KEY POINTS

- Respect is essential to a successful team relationship and is central to achieving good outcomes.
- Respect can be cultivated on an individual, team, and organizational level.
- Uncivil behaviors can be intentional or unintentional but can derail the work of the team and have detrimental effects on patient outcomes.

ACTIVITIES

Activity 1: Role-Play

Read the following brief scripts out loud with another person. Then discuss the questions that follow each script.

SCRIPT 1

Person 1: Ugh, have you seen the new hire? I do not know their name, but they look like they may not have an American accent, if you know what I mean.

Person 2: I hope they don't have a thick accent. If they do I am just going to try and avoid them.

Person 1: I'm going to do the same thing!

Reflection questions:

1. What concepts from the chapter can you identify in this exchange?

2. How could ignoring a team member affect the team as a whole?

3. How could a bystander respond to person 1 and person 2's statements about the new hire in a civil manner?

4. Suggest two to three behaviors or activities that could ease the transition of adding a new member to an already established team.

SCRIPT 2

Person 1: I have been dying to ask you a question since we started working together: Where did you go to college?

Person 2: Why do you ask?

Person 1: Well, for starters you look young, and I have always been impressed by the quality of your work so I was just wondering.

Person 2: Do you ask everyone that question?

Person 1: No. But you appear to be younger than most of our coworkers, so I was curious.

Person 2: It feels as if you are trying to decide if I am qualified for my job.

Reflection questions:

1. What biases, if any, does person 1 demonstrate?

2. How could this interaction affect the team? Include positive and negative outcomes.

3. What are some ways the leader of the team might integrate diversity, equity, and inclusion practices to prevent incivility within the team?

Activity 2: Establishing Ground Rules for the Team

When fostering respect within an interprofessional team it is helpful to establish ground rules or team norms. This activity can be done formally when creating the team, as a team contract, or informally. Before discussing ground rules, team members should reflect on their previous experiences working within a team. Having an idea of team attributes that have and have not led to team success will facilitate the conversation. When developing ground rules for the team consider these factors:

1. What behaviors are most important while working in a group?

2. Are there specific expectations the team members should uphold when communicating with one another?

3. How will decisions be made?

4. How will conflicts be handled?

Activity 3: Team Huddling

Team huddles are meetings to brief the team in preparation for an activity or to check in or regroup during the activity. Team huddles are different from traditional meetings as they require input from all team members. Individuals should discuss what is and is not working well within the team. The team sets the terms of the team huddles, such as the information expected to be shared, who should participate, and where the huddles will occur. Team huddles are meant to be short meetings and can be held as often as necessary based on the team's needs. Utilizing this focused meeting promotes accountability and ensures the team is working toward the same goals.

DISCUSSION QUESTIONS

1. Identify a team that you work with regularly or a team that you have observed working together.

2. Does that team currently use huddles in their team to share information?

    a) If so, does everyone on the team contribute to the huddle? Why or why not?

    b) If not, how might a huddle be incorporated into the team's routine?

3. What are some of the benefits and challenges to using huddles on a team?

4. What steps can you take to make team huddles more effective and to ensure every team member contributes?

REFERENCES

Adams, L. Y., & Maykut, C. A. (2015). Bullying: The antithesis of caring acknowledging the dark side of the nursing profession. *International. Journal of Caring Sciences, 8*(3), 765–773.

American Medical Association. (2016). Code of Medical Ethics. https://code-medical-ethics.ama-assn.org/

American Nurses Association. (2015). Code of Ethics for Nurses. https://www.nursingworld.org/practice-policy/nursing-excellence/ethics/code-of-ethics-for-nurses/

American Nurses Association. (n.d.). Violence, incivility & bullying. *Nursing World.* https://www.nursingworld.org/practice-policy/work-environment/violence-incivility-bullying

American Nurses Association. (2015, July 22). Position statement on incivility, bullying, and workplace violence. *Nursing World.* https://www.nursingworld.org/practice-policy/nursing-excellence/official-position-statements/id/incivility-bullying-and-workplace-violence/

Andersson, L. M., & Pearson, C. M. (1999). Tit for tat? The spiraling effect of incivility in the workplace. *Academy of Management Review, 24*(3), 452–471. https://doi.org/10.5465/AMR.1999.2202131

AORN Staff. (2021, December 3). *4 actions to promote workplace civility.* Association of Perioperative Nurses. https://www.aorn.org/article/2021-12-03-Promote-Workplace-Civility

Bar-David, S. (2018). What's in an eye roll? It is time we explore the role of workplace incivility in healthcare. *Israel Journal of Health Policy Research, 7,* 15. https://doi.org/10.1186/s13584-018-0209-0

Ciocco, M. (2018). *Fast facts on combating nurse bullying, incivility and workplace violence: What nurses need to know in a nutshell.* Springer.

Clark, C. (2017). *Creating and sustaining civility in nursing education* (2nd ed.). Sigma Theta Tau International.

Clark, C. (2019). Fostering a culture of civility and respect in nursing. *Journal of Nursing Regulation, 10*(1), 44–52. https://doi.org/10.1016/S2155-8256(19)30082-1

Ehie, O., Muse, I., Hill, L., & Bastien, A. (2021). Professionalism: Microaggression in the healthcare setting. *Current Opinion in Anesthesiology, 34*(2), 131. https://doi.org/10.1097/ACO.0000000000000966

Fink-Samnick, E. (2015). The new age of bullying and violence in health care: The interprofessional impact. *Professional Case*

Management, 20(4), 165–174; 175–176. https://doi.org/10.1097/NCM.0000000000000099

Fitzgerald, C., & Hurst, S. (2017). Implicit bias in healthcare professionals: A systematic review. *BMC Med Ethics, 18*(1). https://doi.org/10.1186/s12910-017-0179-8

Garibay, J.C. (2014). *Diversity in the classroom.* UCLA Diversity and Faculty Development. https://equity.ucla.edu/wp-content/uploads/2016/06/DiversityintheClassroom2014Web.pdf

Hall, W. J., Chapman, W. V., Lee, K. M., Merino, Y. M., Thomas, T. W., Payne, B. K., Eng, E., Day, S. H., & Coyne-Beasley, T. (2015). Implicit racial/Ethnic bias among health care professionals and its influence on health care outcomes: A systematic review. *American Journal of Public Health, 105*(12), 60–76. https;//doi.org/10.2105/AJPH.2015.302903

Healey, J. (2012). *Respectful relationships.* The Spinney Press.

Heath, M., Williams, E. N., & Wynn, D. (2021). Experiential learning activity to ameliorate workplace bullying. *Journal of Education for Business, 96*(7), 476–483. https://doi.org/10.1080/08832323.2020.1858016

Holsinger, J. W., & Carlton, E. L. (2018). *Leadership for public health: Theory and practice.* Health Administration Press.

Holtschneider, M. E., & Park, C. W. (2021). Addressing blame, shame, bullying, incivility, and microaggression in the interprofessional learning environment: Implications for nursing professional development practitioners. *Journal for Nurses in Professional Development, 37*(1), 54–55.

Houshmand, M., O'Reilly, J., Robinson, S., & Wolff, A. (2012). Escaping bullying: The simultaneous impact of individual and unit-level bullying on turnover intentions. *Human Relations, 65*(7), 901–918. https://doi.org/10.1177/0018726712445100

Hutton, S., & Gates, D. (2008). Workplace incivility and productivity losses among direct care staff. *AAOHN Journal: Official Journal of the American Association of Occupational Health Nurses, 56*(4), 168–175. https://doi.org/10.3928/08910162-20080401-01

Kenney, G. (2014). *Interrupting microaggressions.* College of the Holy Cross, Diversity Leadership & Education.

Kirwan Institute for the Study of Race and Ethnicity (2015). *Understanding implicit bias.* https://kirwaninstitute.osu.edu/implicit-bias-module-series

Limbong, A. (2020, June 9). Microaggressions are a big deal: How to talk them out and when to walk away. *NPR.* https://www.npr.org/2020/06/08/872371063/microaggressions-are-a-big-deal-how-to-talk-them-out-and-when-to-walk-away

Linabary, J. R., & Castro, M. (2021). *Small group communication: Forming & sustaining teams.* Open Textbook Library. https://open.umn.edu/opentextbooks/textbooks/1049

Martin, L. D., & Zadinsky, J. K. (2022). Frequency and outcomes of workplace incivility in healthcare: A scoping review of the literature. *Journal of Nursing Management, 30*(7), 3496–3518. https://doi.org/10.1111/jonm.13783

McLean, K. C., Pasupathi, M., & Syed, M. (2023). Cognitive scripts and narrative identity are shaped by structures of power. *Trends in Cognitive Sciences, 27*(9), 805–813. https://doi.org/10.1016/j.tics.2023.03.006

Merriam-Webster. (2022). Respect. In Merriam-Webster.com dictionary. Retrieved on March 20, 2023, from https://www.merriam-webster.com/dictionary/respect

Okpala, P. (2021). Addressing power dynamics in interprofessional health care teams. *International Journal of Healthcare Management, 14*(4), 1326–1332. https://doi.org/10.1080/20479700.2020.1758894

Parikh, A. K., & Leschied, J. R. (2022). Microaggressions in our daily workplace encounters: A barrier to achieving diversity and inclusion. *Pediatric Radiology, 52*(9), 1719–1723. https://doi.org/10.1007/s00247-022-05307-9

Persily, C. A. (2013). *Team leadership and partnering in nursing and health care*. Springer.

Porath, C., & Pearson, C. (2013). The price of incivility. *Harvard Business Review*. https://hbr.org/2013/01/the-price-of-incivility

Project Implicit. (2011). *Home page*. https://www.projectimplicit.net

Pullon, S. (2008). Competence, respect and trust: Key features of successful interprofessional nurse-doctor relationships. *Journal of Interprofessional Care, 22*(2), 133–147. https://doi.org/10.1080/13561820701795069

Sokol-Hessner, L., Folcarelli, P. H., Annas, C. L., Brown, S. M., Fernandez, L., Roche, S. D., Lee, B. S., Sands, K. E., Atlas, T., Benoit, D. D., Burke, G. F., Butler, T. P., Federico, F., Gandhi, T., Geller, G., Hickson, G. B., Hoying, C., Lee, T. H., Reynolds, M. E., & Rozenblum, R. (2018). A road map for advancing the practice of respect in health care: The results of an interdisciplinary modified Delphi consensus study. *Joint Commission Journal on Quality & Patient Safety, 44*(8), 463–476.

Sue, D. W., Capodilupo, C. M., Torino, G. C., Bucceri, J. M., Holder, A. M. B., Nadal, K. L., & Esquilin, M. (2007). Racial microaggressions in everyday life: Implications for clinical practice. *American Psychologist, 62*(4), 271–286. https://doi.org/10.1037/0003-066X.62.4.271

The Joint Commission. (2021, June). *Quick safety 24: Bullying has no place in health care*. https://www.jointcommission.org/resources/news-and-multimedia/newsletters/newsletters/quick-safety/quick-safety-issue-24-bullying-has-no-place-in-health-care/bullying-has-no-place-in-health-care/#.ZAIW7nbMJeU

The Ohio State University. (n.d.). *Mitigating implicit bias in health care*. https://u.osu.edu/breakingbias/

Woelfle, C. Y. & McCaffrey, R. (2007). Nurse on nurse. *Nursing Forum, 42*(3), 123–131. https://doi.org/10.1111/j.1744-6198.2007.00076.x

CHAPTER 7

Conflict Management

Carol Savrin, DNP, RN, CPNP, R, FNP-BC, FAANP, FNAP, and
Jesse Honsky, DNP, MPH, RN, PHNA-BC

KEY AACN COMPETENCIES, SUB-COMPETENCIES, AND CONCEPTS

Domain 6: Interprofessional Partnerships

Competency 6.1 Communicate in a manner that facilitates a partnership approach to quality care delivery.

- *Entry-Level Sub-Competency 6.1b* Use various communication tools and techniques effectively.
- *Advanced-Level Sub-Competency 6.1l* Demonstrate capacity to resolve interprofessional conflict.

Competency 6.4 Work with other professions to maintain a climate of mutual learning, respect, and shared values.

- *Entry-Level Sub-Competency 6.4c* Engage in constructive communication to facilitate conflict management.
- *Advanced-Level Sub-Competency 6.4h* Manage disagreements, conflicts and challenging conversations among team members.

Concepts for Nursing Practice

- Communication

KEY TERMS

Conflict	Intergroup conflict
Avoiding	Accommodating
Intrapersonal conflict	Intragroup conflict
Competing	Collaborating
Interpersonal conflict	Psychological safety
Compromising	

INTRODUCTION: WHAT IS CONFLICT?

Conflict is a regular occurrence in health care settings and among interprofessional team members. In one survey, 53% of nurses reported that conflict was common or very common in their workplace (Friesen et al., 2009). Conflict occurs among health care professionals (HCP) or between HCPs and patients, or HCPs may have to play a role in conflict management when conflict arises between patients and their family members. The stressful environment of health care contributes to this conflict; for example, HCPs working in pediatric settings report that 73% of end-of-life discussions result in conflict among HCPs (58%) and between HCPs and parents (38%; Archambault-Grenier et al., 2018). While conflict often has a negative connotation, it can have a positive effect on work environments because it supports good decision-making, critical thinking, and innovation (Kim et al., 2015). To be effective leaders, nurses need to understand how conflict may influence teams and organizations in both positive and negative ways and how to address conflict in a constructive manner. This chapter will provide an overview of important concepts in conflict and strategies for managing conflict in interprofessional teams.

Conflict is perceived and defined in many ways. It is often considered a serious disagreement or argument, but it can also be a discrepancy of viewpoints (Borkowski & Meese, 2021). More broadly, conflict is "defined as the internal or external discord that results from differences in ideas, values or feelings between two or more people" (Marquis & Huston, 2021, p. 552). Conflict occurs within and among individuals, groups, and organizations in many different contexts. It can arise when people are required to participate in an activity that does not match their needs or interests, when resources are limited, when there are differences in expectations and preferences, or when they have to rely on others to perform functions and activities of their role (Rahim, 2011).

Three major types of conflict are task conflict, process conflict, and interpersonal conflict (Tannenbaum & Salas, 2021). Task conflict relates to the content and the outcomes of the work. This can be a common source of conflict in an interprofessional team when there are differences of opinion or goals even though the desired outcome may be the same. The conflict occurs over how to get to the outcome, not the outcome itself. For example, a nurse practitioner and physician may have different opinions on the best treatment plan for a patient with diabetes. They both want the same outcome, for the patient to manage their diabetes and avoid future complications from the disease, but they do not agree on the best way to get there. This difference in opinion may stem from a variety of sources. They may have different goals; the nurse practitioner prefers the treatment plan that is more affordable for the patient, and the physician prefers the treatment plan that uses a highly effective but more expensive medication. This also happens in health care when HCPs of different professions use different words to describe the same thing or do not have a shared understanding of the situation. A nurse and a social worker may discuss home-going care but may use different terminology to address the patient's issues. Nurses often talk about medications and return appointments and support personnel. Social workers might talk about support personnel but usually talk about family members and not as much about home health aides. Social workers may also talk about transportation, which the nurse may not identify as a potential issue.

Process conflict is related to the logistics of how the work gets done, for example, the roles and responsibilities of team members or how tasks are assigned. An example of this in health care is when the staff working on the day shift may avoid restocking supplies because "the night shift team is supposed to do that." In this situation, conflict may arise when the staff on night shifts does not have enough supplies readily available, so they perceive the day shift staff as avoiding responsibility; if the supplies are not restocked regularly, everyone assumes that someone else will complete the task. If processes are perceived to be unfair or biased, this can lead to conflict as well. For example, in a hospital unit, there may be a perception that one nurse gets more of their desired days off than others. That can be perceived as favoritism, which can create friction between team members.

Interpersonal conflicts involve personal issues, so the conflict is not about who will do the work and how; it is about how individuals relate to one another. For example, during the monthly clinic staff meeting, a dietician interrupts a PA multiple times as they try to share their opinion about how to improve the referral system to specialty care. The PA perceives this as disrespectful and withdraws from the conversation. In this situation, the conflict revolves more around the behavior of the two people and how they interact. While the conflict is not about the tasks or processes of the work they do, it can still have a negative impact on the work. No matter the source of the conflict, if it is not managed well in interprofessional teams, it leads to poorer patient outcomes in the long run (Bosch & Mansell, 2015).

Conflict is an inevitable part of human interaction and can be positive or negative. If two parties are in conflict and can successfully negotiate and come to a consensus, many times the outcome is better than if the conflict had not occurred. However, this is not an easy process, and it can create great animosity if not handled appropriately (Marquis & Huston, 2021). Conflict challenges us to think differently, to be more creative, to develop a greater understanding, and to search for alternative avenues that are more efficient, more effective, and more productive. If there is negative conflict in a health care setting, generally, the outcome for the patient is worse. When there is conflict within a team on a unit, there is higher turnover in staff, more absenteeism, more stress, and poor productivity (Vandergoot et al., 2018). In addition, this conflict may create an organizational culture of negativity (Dinkin et al., 2013).

SCENARIO 1

The interprofessional team in the pediatric intensive care unit (PICU) was caring for some very ill patients when they received notification that there would be some new patients who would need to be admitted soon. The team working with Kiara, a physician, was caring for one of the extremely ill patients and was responsible for one of the patients who needed to be admitted. Mary was a nurse caring for the severely ill patient and asked the emergency department to wait to transfer the new patient until more staff was available to admit the patient to the PICU. Kiara stormed into the PICU and demanded to know who was responsible for the admission process for her patient and why the patient had not yet been admitted. She stated that the family was very upset and the resident working with her had other things to do and did not have time to wait. Mary tried to explain to Kiara that the current patient had very complex needs that had to be addressed right away. Kiara stormed off saying that her patients were never a top priority for the PICU team. This angry exchange was heard by the rest of the staff and several parents who were in the PICU at the time. This depicts a conflict that created animosity between the physician and the nurse and that also has the potential to impact the other people in the PICU at the time.

Discussion Questions

1. What else would you like to know about this conflict? From Mary's perspective? From Kiara's perspective?
2. How might an interaction like this impact the other members of the interprofessional team? The patients and their parents?
3. How might this interaction impact the culture of the PICU?
4. If you were in either Mary's or Kiaras's position, what might you do differently?
5. How can either Mary or Kiara address the situation now that it has occurred?
6. Imagine you are a nurse manager in this PICU. How would you address the situation now that it has occurred?

Another way to categorize conflict is based on who is involved in the conflict. These categories of conflict include intrapersonal conflict, interpersonal conflict, intergroup conflict, and intragroup conflict (see Figure 7.1; Borkowski & Meese, 2021). Intrapersonal conflict is within one person; after the exchange that occurred in scenario 1 Mary may decide that the conflict in the PICU has impacted the work environment and her life in a negative way and she should consider moving to a different floor; however, she really likes the patient population and loves the challenge of the PICU. Ultimately, she feels torn between staying in the PICU or finding a new position in a more supportive environment.

Interpersonal conflict is what most people think of as conflict, that is, a disagreement or argument between two people like the conflict between Kiara and Mary. Note that this definition is a little different from the description of interpersonal conflict earlier in the chapter. In this context, interpersonal references indicate that the conflict is between two people but does not specify the source of the conflict.

Intergroup conflict is between groups, like teams. What if the emergency department in scenario 1 was too full and did not have room or capacity to keep the patient there? The emergency department team may perceive the request from the PICU to delay the transfer as irresponsible or not in the patient's best interest. This may build resentment between the emergency department team and the PICU team.

Intragroup conflict is within a group or team; after leaving the PICU Kiara meets with the nurse practitioner and resident on her team and begins to complain about the situation. The resident speaks up saying that he agrees with Mary's decision to wait on the admission, and this sparks a debate among the team members.

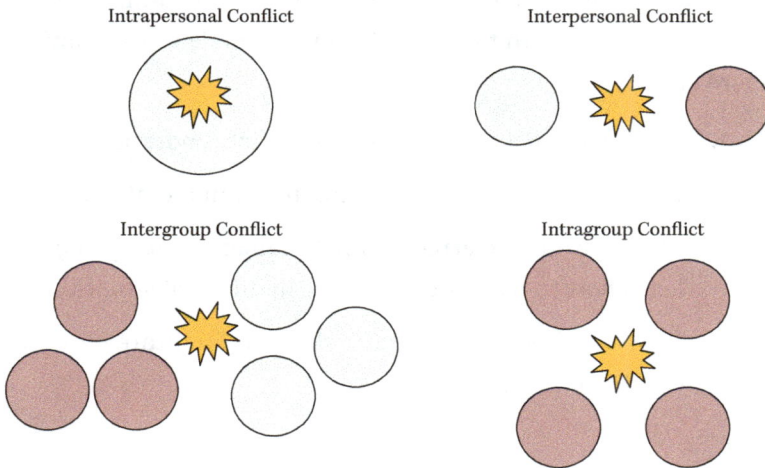

Intrapersonal Conflict

Interpersonal Conflict

Intergroup Conflict

Intragroup Conflict

FIGURE 7.1   Intrapersonal, interpersonal, intergroup, and intragroup conflict.

Understanding the different types and sources of conflict is an important step to understanding how to manage conflict in a manner that supports interprofessional teamwork and collaboration. Nurses interact with many different members of the interprofessional team and thus can play an important role in leading positive conflict management among their team members and in their health care organizations.

APPLICATION TO PRACTICE: HOW DO WE MANAGE CONFLICT?

Conflict management is more than just resolving conflicts and helping teams get along better. It includes creating strategies that are effective for reducing the dysfunction conflict can cause and increasing the positive impacts of conflict with the purpose of improving learning and effectiveness of the team or organization (Borkowski & Meese, 2021; Rahim, 2011; Marquis & Huston 2017). Effective conflict management requires a proactive approach. Interprofessional teams can take steps to set the stage for healthy conflict management to be better prepared for when conflict arises. As an individual on an interprofessional team, there are specific steps you can take to help your team deal with conflict more effectively:

1. Accept and acknowledge that conflict is normal.

2. Foster psychological safety among team members.

3. Identify your preferred conflict management style(s) and learn how to use different styles in different situations.

4. Learn and practice specific skills to facilitate effective conflict management.

Conflict Is Normal

Conflict is a part of normal human interaction that should not be viewed as a sign of failure, and it cannot be ignored or suppressed indefinitely (Tannenbaum & Salas, 2021). In health care settings, conflict is perceived as harmful to the team or even unprofessional, leading to health care professionals avoiding conflict or trying to resolve it too quickly (Eichbaum, 2018). Not only is conflict normal, but it potentially can be beneficial. This requires a shift in perspective from viewing conflict as a problem to be solved, something that should be avoided, or something that only happens in ineffective teams, to viewing it as a resource for learning and innovation (Eichbaum, 2018; Engeström, 2008). For example, if a respiratory therapist mistakenly administers the wrong dose of a medication, this could potentially lead to conflict among the health care team members and potentially even between the team and the patient. Addressing this conflict in a constructive manner can result in the health care team identifying strategies to reduce the chances of others making the same medical error in the future. However, if it is dealt with in a dysfunctional manner it may result in team members being less likely to speak up when an error occurs.

In conjunction with understanding that conflict is normal, acknowledging that conflict may not always be resolved in the first attempt (or at all) helps to set realistic expectations for dealing with conflict. A conflict may take multiple attempts to resolve, or it may simply be an ongoing issue to be managed in a manner that helps the interprofessional team learn and improve their performance. As a member and leader of an interprofessional team, take time to identify if the conflict the team is experiencing is dysfunctional and harmful or, if managed well, it can be a source for learning and improve team effectiveness (Rahim, 2011). Each member of the interprofessional team has a responsibility to address conflict in a respectful and constructive manner.

Fostering Psychological Safety

Another strategy to help promote effective conflict management is to promote psychological safety among team members. Team psychological safety is "a shared belief that the team is safe for interpersonal risk" (Edmondson, 1999, p. 154). Simply put, this means that all members of the team feel comfortable speaking up when they have concerns without fear of embarrassment, rejection, or punishment from their team members because there is mutual respect and trust among team members (Edmondson,

1999). Psychological safety does not mean that the team always gets along and never disagrees with each other or that team members do not hold each other accountable. In fact, a team with strong psychological safety will encourage respectful disagreement and speak up when a team member is not carrying their weight or makes a mistake, though they will do so in a respectful manner. This is important in health care as team members can help each other make good decisions or avoid making errors that could harm patients.

The concept of psychological safety feels intuitive to many people, and many health care providers agree that creating a safe environment to speak up will improve patient safety. A challenge arises in translating that understanding into action. Many people struggle to find the "right" words or actions for difficult situations and conversations; this is not as intuitive. Table 7.1 provides some tips to help foster psychological safety among teams and examples of words or actions an individual can use in the health care setting.

TABLE 7.1   **Tips for Fostering Psychological Safety in Health Care Teams**

Tips for Peers and Leaders	Examples of Words or Actions
Thank people for offering their point of view: This is particularly important when you disagree with them. It reinforces that speaking up is expected in your team and that it is safe to offer a dissenting view.	"Thank you for sharing your perspective on issues we are having with the clinic schedule. We need to hear from everyone on the team to try to understand this problem better, even if we have different opinions on how to fix it."
Summarize what other people have said: Convey that you "get it." This tells teammates that you are listening to them and that their perspective matters.	"It sounds like you are frustrated with the new admission checklist; it is too cumbersome, and you feel like it is making your job more difficult."

Tips for Peers and Leaders	Examples of Words or Actions
Be careful about your facial expressions: When you roll your eyes or look "pained," your face may convey that the person is incompetent or pushy. That can not only shut them down but may squelch the other team members too.	Body language is important in communication. Be mindful of your facial expressions to ensure they are congruent with the message you want to convey. This will help to build trust with your teammates and your patients.
Focus on "what's right," not "who's right": You don't need to win every disagreement. It is easier to generate innovative ideas and engage in creative discussion when you feel like you must defend your position at all costs.	"Our team has different ideas on how to improve our referrals for mental health services. How are these proposed solutions going to impact patient care?"
Don't tolerate a teammate saying disparaging things about another teammate: When a teammate is criticized behind their back, other teammates will wonder, "Is anyone saying bad things about me too?" and "Would my teammates stick up for me?"	"You sound like you are frustrated with Juan's handling of that situation with the patient. In my experience, Juan is usually really thoughtful. Have you talked directly to him about your concerns?"
Tips for Leaders	**Application to Health Care**
Admit that you don't know something, don't understand something, or made a mistake: When a leader does this, it makes it much easier for everyone else on the team to do so too.	"I am not familiar with the new prescribing guidelines. Can you help me understand them better?"
Keep an eye on how often team members speak up, voice dissent, provide feedback, ask questions, admit they don't know something or made a mistake, seek assistance, and try out new ideas: These are the behaviors exhibited in psychologically safe teams, so consider this pulse check. If your team isn't doing these enough, talk with team members one on one to find out why.	"I noticed you haven't said much during morning rounds over the past couple of weeks. Is there something that is keeping you from speaking up?"

(Continued)

Tips for Leaders	Application to Health Care
Ask a team member to share their thoughts and opinions—and respond respectfully when they do: Some people, particularly junior team members, need encouragement to speak up. When they do so, the reaction they get will determine if they do so again.	"Greta, you have had experience in the past working at a community health center. What do you think is important for us to think about as we plan to expand our clinic services?"
Be clear about non-negotiables and negotiables: What can't be changed and everything else for which their input is valued. When the team knows which topics are "off limits" and which decisions can't be changed, they are less likely to bring them up. And later, if you need to redirect the discussion away from those issues, they will understand why you are doing so.	"Our hospital system is adopting a new electronic health record (EHR), and the vendor has already been selected. While we can't change the EHR or when it will be implemented in our unit, what can we do to make sure the transition is as seamless as possible?"
Focus more attention on what can be learned from a mistake ("Do differently next time") and less on assigning blame ("You really messed up this time"): A learning-oriented focus allows people to acknowledge their mistakes and ask questions without feeling threatened.	"Now that we see there is a problem in the medication administration workflow, what can we do to make sure this mistake doesn't happen again?"

Source: Adapted from Tips for Peers and Leaders and Tips for Leaders *by Tannenbaum & Salas (2021, pp. 71–72).*

Conflict Management Styles

Once conflict arises, there are a variety of ways to manage it. There is not one style that should be used for all conflicts. In fact, understanding different modes of handling conflict and when to use them appropriately is an important skill for working with an interprofessional team. Some of the most well-known conflict-handling modes are described by Thomas and Kilman (1974); the styles are avoiding, competing, compromising, accommodating, and collaborating. These five modes sit along two dimensions: assertiveness and cooperativeness. Assertiveness focuses on resolving the conflict to meet your needs or concerns, and cooperativeness focuses on resolving the conflict to meet the needs or concerns of others. These dimensions progress along a spectrum with the conflict-handling modes (see Figure 7.2).

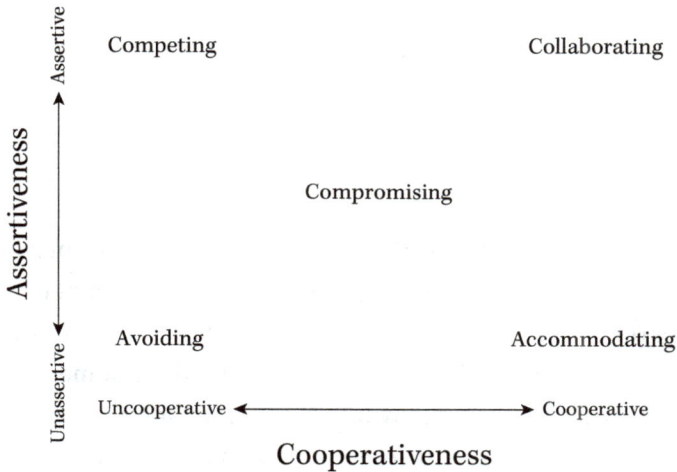

FIGURE 7.2 Thomas and Kilman's conflict-handling modes and dimensions.

SCENARIO 2

Jean, a nurse, is frustrated with Mark, the social worker assigned to the orthopedic floor. Many of Jean's patients go to physical therapy (PT) off the floor, and the transport team always comes for them at about 8:30 a.m., after breakfast. Mark arrives on the floor most days at 8:00 or 8:30. When Mark meets with patients he often needs to talk with them for an extended amount of time. Mark has been told to find out who is scheduled for PT so that he can plan to see those patients later in the day after their therapy sessions. Mark did not check the schedule today, and this is the third time this week that the patient Mark was with missed the PT time because transport left while they were talking. Jean, while frustrated, simply goes about her work, asks transport to come back, and calls the PT department to reschedule. On several occasions they were not able to reschedule.

Discussion Questions

1. What style is Jean using here?
2. What other options might there be?
3. How might the situation be improved? Think of as many options as possible.
4. As you read on, return to this scenario and see if other ideas arise.

AVOIDING

Avoiding is both unassertive and uncooperative. Generally, it can have a negative impact on the health care team because it leaves others feeling frustrated and the conflict is never addressed or resolved (Borkowski & Meese, 2021). There are some circumstances when avoiding may be appropriate, for example if the issue at hand is minor, if someone needs to step away to calm down, or if the situation is threatening (Kilmann, 2018; Rahim, 2011). Ultimately, avoiding should not be an individual's or team's primary strategy to handle conflict.

In scenario 2, Jean appears to be relying on avoiding the conflict instead of addressing it directly with Mark. How might using this strategy impact Jean and Mark's relationship as team members? How might it impact Jean in the future?

COMPETING

Competing is assertive and uncooperative. When using competing to manage conflict, individuals put their needs or ideas first and push to "win" the conflict. This can be harmful to a team, as those on the "losing" side of the conflict may feel ignored or disrespected, and ultimately it may erode psychological safety and trust between team members. Individuals using this form of conflict management may leverage their power in order to win, such as their formal position (team lead or manager) or ability to argue (Kilmann, 2018). As with avoiding, there may be certain circumstances when competing may be appropriate, for example in an emergency and when the wrong decision could cause harm, when an individual needs to stand up for their rights, or if the issue is minor. Individuals who work in formal leadership roles may also need to use a competing strategy when an unpopular decision needs to be made (Borkowski & Meese, 2021; Kilmann, 2018; Rahim, 2011).

Imagine if, in scenario 2 Jean and Mark took a competing approach to address the conflict. What might the conversation around the conflict look like? What might the outcome of the conflict look like? How might this impact the team and the patients?

COMPROMISING

Compromising is moderate in assertiveness and cooperativeness. It tends to work well when the team members involved are equally powerful, the differing goals of the team members do not overlap, and a resolution needs to be found relatively quickly (Kilmann, 2018; Rahim, 2011). While finding compromise is often viewed as a positive outcome of conflict management, it does have downsides. For example, individuals from both parties may walk away from the conflict feeling unsatisfied because they had to give something up, and too much reliance on compromising to handle conflict may create more problems because the real issues causing the conflict are never fully explored or addressed. Finally, while a proposed solution may be a compromise, it may not be the best solution to the problem at hand (Borkowski & Meese, 2021).

If Jean and Mark were to approach their conflict using compromise, what circumstances would need to be in place to help them be successful? What circumstances might indicate that compromise may not make sense for this particular situation?

ACCOMMODATING

Accommodating is unassertive and cooperative. It is different from compromising in that when accommodating only one party gives up something in order to resolve the conflict. It is essentially the opposite of competing (Kilmann, 2018). Accommodating requires an individual to ignore their own concerns or needs to satisfy others. Generally, accommodating is not an effective style to use on a regular basis. When individuals use accommodation too frequently, they may be seen as weak or submissive (Borkowski & Meese, 2021). In addition, it is not appropriate to use it when the other party in the conflict is wrong or unethical (Rahim, 2011). In a team, if accommodation is used too frequently the team may never truly address the conflict, and those who accommodate may begin to feel resentful because they have given up more than others. Some individuals may choose accommodation because they do not feel they have power in the situation or feel intimidated. On the other hand, used sparingly accommodation can be a way to demonstrate generosity, or if the issue is relatively small accommodating may help to build goodwill and support in the long term (Borkowski & Meese, 2021; Kilmann, 2018).

What might accommodating look like from Jean's perspective in scenario 2? What about Mark's perspective? What are the pros and cons of this approach in the situation described?

COLLABORATING

Collaborating is both assertive and cooperative. In many ways collaborating is the ideal conflict management strategy for an interprofessional team. It is the opposite of avoiding in that it requires team members to engage with each other to better understand the source of the conflict, including the underlying needs and wants of the individuals involved (Kilmann, 2018). It is different from compromise in that the resolution benefits all involved and no one feels they had to make a trade-off in order to resolve the conflict. For collaboration to work effectively, team members must have psychological safety so they can share their thoughts and ideas with each, regardless of their roles and perceived hierarchies. There must also be interdependence among the team members, and they must understand how their roles and goals are related to each other. Finally, collaboration takes time; there should be sufficient organizational support to work through conflict using this strategy (Borkowski & Meese, 2021; Winder, 2003). Collaboration is also beneficial in complex situations, as it provides an opportunity to share different ideas and perspectives to find creative solutions to the problems causing the conflict. While collaboration is needed for an interprofessional team to resolve conflict effectively, there are situations when it may not be needed or appropriate, for example in emergency situations when a decision is needed quickly or if the problem is simple and does not require time to make a collaborative decision (Rahim, 2011).

Imagine if you were Jean. How would you approach the conflict with Mark in a collaborative manner? What questions would you ask? What additional information do you need to know? What information do you think Jean should share? Who else might need to join the conversation?

Conflict management is not a one-size-fits-all approach, and understanding how to best apply each of the modes takes intentional practice and can be learned over time. An important step in this is understanding your own preferences for conflict management strategies and reflecting on how you might be using them appropriately and inappropriately. Understanding your preferred conflict management style is helpful when approaching a difficult situation. Activity 1 at the end of this chapter provides information about the U.S. Institute of Peace (n.d.) conflict styles assessment, free online. Complete the assessment and reflection questions to gain a better understanding of your preferred conflict style(s) and get started in this process.

Conflict Management Skills

The skills and knowledge one needs to address conflict effectively align with the skills and knowledge that are expected of nurses in other areas of their practice, such as communication, emotional intelligence, and respect. Often these concepts are applied to how nurses take care of patients; however, they are just as important to how nurses interact with their colleagues. Nurses must take time to learn and practice the skills needed to navigate conflict with their peers, other professionals, and patients. While every situation cannot be re-created in a classroom or lab for practice, learning about, reflecting on, and practicing skills can help you feel more prepared as you transition into your role on the clinical team as a member and leader. Learning conflict management skills will help nurses and other HCPs address conflict in the following ways competently:

- managing conflict between different health care team members
- managing conflicts brought about during transitions of care between teams
- effectively negotiating and managing conflict among patients, families and the health care team
- coaching others in conflict management (Fahy et al., 2021)

TIPS FOR WORKING THROUGH CONFLICT

Communication is key in managing conflict. The most important aspect of communication is listening, which is more than being quiet while someone else is talking; in order to listen, particularly in a situation of conflict, one must put aside all distractions—no phone, no computer, and no other distractions from other people. This means that if one is to have a successful discussion about a topic of conflict, whether with one other person if the conflict is personal or as a facilitator and there are two other people, there should be a separate space, and privacy should be maintained. One must put aside internal "self-talk," such as saying negative things to yourself about the situation or making assumptions about the people involved, and keep an open mind. When one is in a situation trying to resolve conflict, the question "why" can create animosity. When dealing with conflict, try to remove that word from the conversation.

Some of the important points to keep in mind when working to resolve conflict are the following:

- Separate people from the issue.
- Focus on the issue.
- Focus on the best alternative for all.
- Brainstorm.
- Insist that you deal with objective data and remove emotions from the table (Borkowski & Meese, 2021; Dinkin et al., 2013; Fisher et al., 2011).

Think of a conflict you have observed or experienced; this can be a conflict in any setting, at work, school, clinical, or other locations. Reflect on the following questions:

1. How would you separate the people from the issue in the conflict? What is the issue?
2. Once you identify the issue, brainstorm a situation in which the outcome would benefit everyone involved.
3. When thinking about this conflict, identify the objective data to focus on and some of the emotions that the individuals involved might experience.

When encountering conflict, it may be difficult to start the conversation or find the right words. One tool to help with this is called DESC: describe, express, suggest, consequences (Agency for Health Care Research and Quality, 2023). DESC can be used to manage different types of conflict. It follows a four-step process:

1. *Describe* the specific situation or behavior using concrete data.

2. *Express* how the situation makes you feel or what your concerns are.

3. *Suggest* other alternatives, try to reach agreement.

4. *Consequences should be stated* in terms of impact on the patient or team goals; work toward consensus.

The idea is very similar to the tips for working through conflict: Focus on I statements, not you statements; focus on win-win end points; focus on what is right, not who is right.

Nurses can use many different strategies to navigate conflict. One can negotiate, or there can be arbitration through an outside person. Negotiation is the facilitation of trying to reach agreement between two parties who disagree. An arbitrator is often the person in the middle with no vested interest in either side who facilitates the negotiation. Harvard Law School (2014) provides training materials online to help individuals learn more about negotiation (Fisher et al., 2011).

SCENARIO 3

Pat is the nurse who has been caring for Martha for several weeks. Martha is 85 years old and while surgery had been done, she did not appear to be any better than she was when she was admitted. Her daughters visited every day, and Martha was getting more disoriented and often did not recognize them. After one particularly stressful visit, Pat decided to discuss a do not attempt to resuscitate (DNAR) order with the daughters. Pat observed that Martha was not improving and the daughters were more and more distraught on each visit. When the physician learned what had occurred, the physician did not discuss the issue with Pat, and the physician escalated it to nursing administration and indicated that Pat had overstepped his boundaries. The physician told the nursing administration that Martha had a condition that was curable and that eventually she would improve.

Discussion Questions

1. This has been escalated to the nursing administration; what might the supervisor do here?
2. How might this have been handled differently?
3. Might the situation have been avoided? If so, how?
4. What styles are the people here using to address the conflict?
5. Is the supervisor called on to arbitrate? Negotiate?

Unit or Organizational Conflict for Advanced Nurses

In any organization, the interactions are not only between individuals but often between hospital units or organizations. That means that when conflict occurs, it is between groups of people. Those groups of people may have differences, as individuals do, in values, goals, and resources. Often an issue between units or organizations is power. It may be perceived that one unit has more power than another, and frequently that is the result of available resources. If the cardiovascular unit, for example, brings in a lot of money to the hospital, it may have more power and resources, which can create conflict. To maintain the efficient functioning of the cardiovascular unit, more staff may be reserved to work there, while other units may have to go through a lengthy process to request staff when more is needed. This may cause frustration and build resentment between departments in the hospital. In the organizational system, money often leads to power, and power can be misused or at best misunderstood.

There are multiple types of power, and each can create conflict. Positional power, also called legitimate power, is the power of an individual because of the relative position and duties they hold within an organization. Legitimate power is formal authority delegated to person in that position or role, such as a manager or chief executive officer (CEO). Referent power is the power or ability of individuals to attract and inspire others; often, these people have charisma. Expert power is an individual's power deriving from the skills or expertise of the person and the organization's needs for those skills and expertise. Reward power depends on the ability of the power wielder to confer valued material rewards; parents are an example of this type of power. Coercive power is the application of negative influences. It includes the ability to demote or withhold other rewards. Coercive power may lie with a supervisor who can grant time off or approve vacation time (Borkowski & Meese, 2021).

Powerful people are more proactive and more likely to speak up, make the first move, and lead negotiation (Berdahl & Martorana, 2006). Individuals can also use influence and knowledge to exert power. For example, if a person is a trusted colleague of the CEO of an organization, they may have the power to influence the CEO's decisions. Or if a person serves on a planning committee for the design of a new unit, they have power because they have knowledge of what is being discussed for the new unit. This sort of power is often discussed within the U.S. legislature in that legislators have knowledge that may influence the stock market before the majority of people have that knowledge, which thus creates potential improper selling or buying of stocks (Borkowski & Meese, 2021).

Another area in which there can be conflict within an organization is with poor communications or unclear expectations. If the people working on a unit do not understand what is expected of them, conflict is going to arise either within the unit or between units. That conflict can then be used to clarify expectations and improve communication. Sometimes there are written policies that need to be revised, and sometimes there are unwritten expectations that need to be included in the official policies.

When there is conflict between units or organizations, the manager or supervisor is often asked to step up and lead the way. The manager or supervisor should not try to solve the issue unilaterally. That will likely lead to further conflict in the future as people will not believe that they have had input. The manager should arbitrate or negotiate. Generally, it is crucial to have meetings with as many participants in the unit as possible to brainstorm ideas and gather feedback. Then the manager can negotiate or arbitrate a potential solution that is acceptable to most people in the unit or the organization. When a leader is a negotiator, that person needs to look to the future, not perseverate on the past, keep an open mind, watch for aggression, and be careful of insincere flattery. Insincere flattery lulls others into complacency and can erode trust. Engaging as many people in the unit or organization as possible to have input into the solution will help create the best outcome for everyone involved (Lundin et al., 2000).

SCENARIO 4

Jean is an NP working in an internal medicine practice in a large hospital organization. She has been there for 3 years. Three other NPs, two PAs, and three physicians work with her at the internal medicine practice. Since she joined the practice, there has been half a week allotted to administration time. That time is for the providers to return phone calls from patients or other providers, contact insurance companies if needed, follow up on lab tests and external referrals, and review their patient panel to ensure patients followed through on recommendations and were seen appropriately. That time is always filled with these activities. Last week a memo from the hospital organization indicated that the outpatient facilities were not bringing in as much revenue as needed, so the administration time was being eliminated. All of those tasks still needed to be done, but now the providers would have to do them during their lunch break or after hours. Jean works three 12-hour days and doing those activities at 8 o'clock at night is not possible; the other providers, laboratories, and pharmacies are not open that late.

She will have to do all those activities instead of lunch. The other providers are just as frustrated as Jean and begin to complain regularly. After several conversations, they start planning how to get the administration time reinstated.

1. What might be a plan to address this issue?
2. Who should potentially do the ask?
3. Who has power in this situation?
4. What kind of power do they have and why?
5. Who do the providers go to at this point?
6. How should they frame their request?
7. What is necessary for this negotiation?

CONCLUSION

Conflict in health care presents in a variety of ways. Conflict can occur between HCPs, or it can occur between the provider and the patient or the patient's family. The stressful environment of health care often leads to conflict. Not all conflict is problematic; some can promote growth and innovation. Conflict management skills can be learned and must be practiced. Nurses can play a valuable role in leading conflict management in their teams and in their organizations. To do this, nurses must understand why conflict occurs, the role of psychological safety, and different conflict management styles and strategies.

KEY POINTS

- Conflict is normal and, if managed well, can help an interprofessional team learn from each other and improve their performance.
- Psychological safety is essential in developing a positive environment for healthy conflict management.

- Individuals may use different conflict management styles when dealing with conflict; some styles are more effective than others.
- Nurses and other health care professionals should not avoid conflict; they should learn to develop the skills to manage conflict appropriately, such as communication, negotiation, and arbitration.
- Power can play a role in creating or managing conflict. Understanding the types of power leveraged in an organization can help you to understand how to manage conflict effectively.

ACTIVITIES

Activity 1: Conflict Styles Assessment

Complete the U.S. Institute of Peace's (n.d.) conflict styles assessment online. This assessment is based on the Thomas Kilmann Conflict Mode Instrument (Thomas & Kilman, 1974) and identifies five different conflict styles: compromiser, problem solver, accommodator, competer, and avoider. After completing the assessment, review the results and reflect on the following questions:

1. According to your results, which conflict style(s) are you more likely to use when you encounter conflict? What are some situations when it may be beneficial to use this style?

2. Which style(s) are you least likely to use? What are some situations when it may be beneficial to use this style?

3. What is a style that you would like to incorporate more into your interactions with other health professionals? What are some concrete steps you can take to do this?

4. How might someone's individual experience, social status, or role in the health care team impact how they approach conflict?

Ryan, a nurse practitioner, went into an exam room to see a patient named Jim. As Ryan was reviewing the EHR, he noticed that the vital signs from today's visit were not recorded. As one of Jim's major problems was hypertension, it was not possible to proceed without the vital signs. Ryan stormed out of the exam room, leaving the door open. He found the medical assistant, Shelley, who usually does vital signs in the hallway. Ryan proceeded to shout at Shelley saying, "How do you expect me to do my job and stay on time if you cannot even put the vital signs into the chart?" Shelley tried to explain that she had been tied up with another patient and that someone else had done the vital signs, but she did not know whom. Ryan kept telling her that it was her job and then walked down the hall shouting "Who is the incompetent person who did the vital signs on Jim and did not record them? How do any of you expect me to do my job?" On his way down the hall Ryan passed several patients, a clinic nurse, and the receptionist.

a.   What is the issue?

b.   What is the issue from each person's point of view?

c.   What emotions are evidenced here?

d.   How might the patients perceive this interaction?

e.   What would be the best possible outcome for each role?

f.   Brainstorm some ways to address the situation.

g.   What would you say to Ryan or Shelley in this situation to help manage the conflict?

Think about a conflict you experienced or observed. This could be a conflict in any setting, at work, school, in health care, or other settings.

1. Describe the conflict. What were the most important issues in the conflict?

2. What type of conflict styles did you use or see other people use?

3. Do you think that conflict was managed well? Why or why not?

REFERENCES

Agency for Health Care Research and Quality. (2023). *Tool: DESC*. https://www.ahrq.gov/teamstepps-program/curriculum/mutual/tools/desc.html

American Colleges of Nursing. (2021). *The essentials: Core competencies for professional nursing education.* https://www.aacnnursing.org/AACN-Essentials/Download

Archambault-Grenier, M.-A., Roy-Gagnon, M.-H., Gauvin, F., Doucet, H., Humbert, N., Stojanovic, S., Payot, A., Fortin, S., Janvier, A., & Duval, M. (2018). Survey highlights the need for specific interventions to reduce frequent conflicts between healthcare professionals providing paediatric end-of-life care. *Acta Paediatrica, 107*(2), 262–269. https://doi.org/10.1111/apa.14013

Berdahl, J. L., & Martorana, P. (2006). Effects of power on emotion and expression during a controversial group discussion. *European Journal of Social Psychology, 36*(4), 497–509. https://doi.org/10.1002/ejsp.354

Borkowski, N., & Meese, K. A. (2021). *Organizational behavior in health care* (4th ed.). Jones & Bartlett Learning.

Bosch, B., & Mansell, H. (2015). Interprofessional collaboration in health care: Lessons to be learned from competitive sports. *Canadian Pharmacists Journal / Revue Des Pharmaciens Du Canada, 148*(4), 176–179. https://doi.org/10.1177/1715163515588106

Dinkin, S., Filner, B., & Maxwell, L. (2013). *The exchange strategy for managing conflict in health care: How to defuse emotions and create solutions when the stakes are high.* McGraw-Hill.

Edmondson, A. (1999). Psychological safety and learning behavior in work teams. *Administrative Science Quarterly, 44*(2), 350–383. https://doi.org/10.2307/2666999

Eichbaum, Q. (2018). Collaboration and teamwork in the health professions: Rethinking the role of conflict. *Academic Medicine, 93*(4), 574–580. https://doi.org/10.1097/ACM.0000000000002015

Engeström, Y. (2008). *From teams to knots: Activity-theoretical studies of collaboration and learning at work.* Cambridge University Press.

Fahy, A. S., Mueller, C., & Fecteau, A. (2021). Conflict resolution and negotiation in pediatric surgery. *Seminars in Pediatric Surgery, 30*(5), 151100. https://doi.org/10.1016/j.sempedsurg.2021.151100

Fisher, R., Ury, W., & Patton, B. (2011). *Getting to yes.* Penguin.

Friesen, M. A., Vernell, D., Osborne, J., & Rosenkranz, A. (2009). Nurses, perceptions of conflict in the workplace: Results of the Center for American Nurses. *Nurses First, 2,* 12–16.

Harvard Law School. (2014). *Negotiation strategies and negotiation techniques to help you become a better negotiator.* https://www.pon.harvard.edu/freemium/negotiation-skills-negotiation-strategies-and-negotiation-techniques-to-help-you-become-a-better-negotiator/

Kilmann, R. H. (2018, June 1). *Take the Thomas-Kilmann conflict mode instrument (TKI).* Kilmann Diagnostics. https://kilmanndiagnostics.com/overview-thomas-kilmann-conflict-mode-instrument-tki/

Kim, W. S., Nicotera, A. M., & McNulty, J. (2015). Nurses' perceptions of conflict as constructive or destructive. *Journal of Advanced Nursing, 71*(9), 2073–2083. https://doi.org/10.1111/jan.12672

Lundin, S. C., Paul, H., & Christensen, J. (2000). *Fish! A remarkable way to boost morale and improve results.* Hyperion.

Marquis, B. L., & Huston, C. J. (2021). *Leadership roles and management functions in nursing: Theory and application* (10th ed.). Wolters Kluwer.

Rahim, M. A. (2011). *Managing conflict in organizations* (4th ed.). Routledge.

Tannenbaum, S. I., & Salas, E. (2021). *Teams that work: The seven drivers of team effectiveness.* Oxford University Press.

Thomas, K. W., & Kilman, R. H. (1974). *Thomas-Kilman conflict mode instrument.* Xicom.

U.S. Institute of Peace. (n.d.). *Conflict styles assessment.* https://www.usip.org/public-education-new/conflict-styles-assessment

Vandergoot, S., Sarris, A., Kirby, N., & Ward, H. (2018). Exploring undergraduate students' attitudes towards interprofessional learning, motivation-to-learn, and perceived impact of learning conflict resolution skills. *Journal of Interprofessional Care, 32*(2), 211–219. https://doi.org/10.1080/13561820.2017.1383975

Winder, R. (2003). Organizational dynamics and development. *Futurics, 27*(1/2), 5–30.

CREDIT

CHAPTER 8

Personal Health, Resilience, and Well-Being

Deborah Lindell, DNP, MSN, RN, CNE, ANEF, FAAN, and Beverly Capper, DNP, MSN, RNC-NIC

KEY AACN COMPETENCIES, SUB-COMPETENCIES, AND CONCEPTS

Domain 10: Personal, Professional, and Leadership Development

Competency 10.1 Demonstrate a commitment to personal health and well-being.

- *Entry-Level Sub-Competency 10.1a* Demonstrate healthy self-care behaviors that promote wellness and resiliency.

- *Entry-Level Sub-Competency 10.1b* Manage conflict between personal and professional responsibilities.

- *Advanced-Level Sub-Competency 10.1c* Contribute to an environment that promotes self-care, personal health, and well-being.

- *Advanced-Level Sub-Competency 10.1d* Evaluate the workplace environment to determine level of health and well-being.

Concepts
- Communication
- Diversity, equity, and inclusion

KEY TERMS

Health	Mindfulness
Self-care	Systems-based practice
Healthy lifestyle	Resilience
Stress management	Wellness and well-being

INTRODUCTION: HEALTH AND WELL-BEING FOR NURSES

You can't pour from an empty cup. Take care of yourself first.
—Norm Kelly, Twitter, January 3, 2018

Nurses do it all! They make critical decisions, advocate for their patients, implement skilled procedures, collaborate with the health care team, and more, all through compassionate, healing relationships and the nursing process. Beyond individual patients, nurses provide care to families, communities, and populations, and they are educators, managers, and leaders within nursing and interprofessional teams. Regardless of the practice setting, nurses are challenged by the ever-increasing acuity of patients and the intensity of their work environments (American Nurses Association [ANA], 2015).

As a result, today's nurses often experience suboptimal personal health and well-being, compassion fatigue, burnout, and moral distress that may lead to high turnover rates or leaving the nursing profession altogether. Table 8.1 provides definitions of compassion fatigue, burnout, and moral distress (American Association of Critical Care Nurses [AACN], 2020). While they are distinct types of distress, compassion fatigue and moral distress are two of many factors that can lead to burnout.

TABLE 8.1   Differences Between Moral Distress, Burnout, and Compassion Fatigue

Moral Distress	Burnout	Compassion Fatigue
When one knows the right thing to do but constraints, conflict, dilemmas, or uncertainty make it nearly impossible to pursue the right course of action.	Physical, mental, and emotional exhaustion caused by workplace stress, leading to disengagement and depersonalization.	Physical, mental, and emotional weariness related to caring for those in significant pain or emotional distress.

In 2015, the ANA acknowledged "significant changes, sometimes perceived as barriers, to achieving healthy work environments that support and promote the best patient care and the (personal) health and well-being of the nurse" (p. 21). These issues accelerated during the COVID-19 pandemic (American Nurses Foundation [ANF], 2023).

Yet, nurses also experience joy and contentment with their practice, especially "making a difference in people's lives" (Medscape, 2022, slide 4). When asked, nurses can recall gratifying encounters with patients that reinforced their commitment to nursing as a helping profession. What can be done to address the demands of nursing practice, prevent burnout and turnover, and enhance nurses' satisfaction? A multiprong, multilevel approach is needed, and the urgency could not be greater! Many reports have addressed this priority, such as *The Future of Nursing 2020–2030: Charting a Path to Achieve Health Equity*. In Chapter 10 they note,

> Nurses' health and well-being are affected by the demands of their workplace, and in turn, their well-being affects their work and the people they care for. As it has in so many other areas, COVID-19 has imposed new challenges for the well-being of nurses. But it also has offered opportunities to give nurses' well-being the attention it deserves and to address the systems, structures, and policies that create workplace hazards and stresses that lead to burnout, fatigue, and poor physical and mental health. if nurses are not supported in maintaining their physical, emotional, and mental well-being and integrity, their ability to serve and support patients, families, and communities will be compromised. ... Policymakers, employers of nurses, nursing schools, nurse leaders, professional associations, and nurses themselves all have a role in ensuring the well-being

of the nursing workforce." (National Academies of Sciences, Engineering, and Medicine [NASEM], 2021, p. 301)

This chapter will present multilevel strategies, from the individual to systems, to promote nurses' health and well-being by supporting their personal self-care. Self-care is "the act of attending to one's physical or mental health, generally without medical or other professional consultation" (AACN, 2021, p. 64). It includes meaningful activities that make us feel good about ourselves, our futures, and our lives. There are no limits to self-care. It comes down to the quality, intention, and proactiveness of the action. Table 8.2 provides a few examples of personal self-care. We'll discuss more later.

TABLE 8.2   **Examples of Feel-Good Self-Care Practices**

Do something that energizes you.
Call a friend or family member.
Create a gratitude list.
Declutter and get organized.

Important Definitions

This chapter provides nurses with tools to commit to personal self-care and help improve health and well-being in their work environment. To get started, we identified definitions of the key terms and concepts used throughout the chapter, as many are sometimes used interchangeably or have different meanings to different people.

Health: "Health is more than the absence of disease; it is a resource that allows people to realize their aspirations, satisfy their needs and to cope with the environment in order to live a long, productive, and fruitful life" (Centers for Disease Control and Prevention [CDC], 2018).

Healthy lifestyle: "A way of living that lowers the risk of being seriously ill or dying early. Scientific studies have identified certain types of behavior that contribute to the development of noncommunicable diseases and early death" (AACN, 2021, p. 59).

Mindfulness: "The basic human ability to be fully present, aware of where we are and what we're doing, and not overly reactive or overwhelmed by what's going on around us" (Mindful, 2023, para. 3).

Resilience: "The ability to survive and thrive in the face of adversity. Resilience can be developed and internalized ... to improve retention and reduce burnout (AACN, 2021, p. 63).

Self-care: "The act of attending to one's physical or mental health, generally without medical or other professional consultation" (AACN, 2021, p. 64)

Stress management: "A range of strategies to help better deal with stress and difficulty (adversity) (AACN, 2021, p. 65).

Systems-based practice: "An analytical tool and a way of viewing the world, which can make caregiving and change efforts more successful. The focus is on understanding the interdependencies of a system or series of systems and the changes identified to improve care that can be made and measured in the system" (AACN, 2021, p. 66)

Wellness and well-being: "A state of being marked by emotional stability (e.g., coping effectively with life and creating satisfying relationships) and physical health (e.g., recognizing the need for physical activity, healthy foods, and sleep" (AACN, 2021, p. 66).

APPLICATION TO PRACTICE: HOW CAN NURSES CARE FOR THEMSELVES?

This section discusses how nurses can practice personal self-care to promote their own health, well-being, and resilience in their work environment. Self-care is a type of behavior. We know that an individual needs the necessary knowledge and skills to perform a particular behavior successfully. However, knowledge and skills aren't enough. One's attitudes toward the behavior are also important. A positive attitude toward an activity and one's self-efficacy, the belief that one can do the activity, increase the likelihood one will commit to the activity and prioritize it in their life (Pender, 2011). Throughout this section, we will incorporate ways to enhance your attitude about self-care.

Self-care is a form of self-love that helps us maintain physical and emotional fitness and promote personal resilience. For nurses in particular, responsibility for self-care is a standard of ethical nursing practice (ANA, 2005) and a strategy to help prevent and reduce the effects of today's high-demand health care environment on our health and well-being.

Health and Well-Being

Health is more than not being ill; it includes "physical, mental and social well-being" (AACN, 2021, p. 65). One of nursing's core values is that we view persons holistically. Holistic, an abstract term, means viewing and valuing something or someone as more than the sum of the parts. While nurses focus on the health of humans, a car is a good example of something that is holistic. You can lay out all the parts of a car, but it is not a means of transportation for work or recreation until it is assembled, fueled, and licensed. The same idea applies to a band, orchestra, or an arch of stones (see Figure 8.1).

Thus, nurses provide holistic care, "the integration of mind-body-emotion-spirit-sexual-cultural-energetic-environmental principles and modalities to promote health, increase well-being, and actualize human potential" (ANA, 2015, p. 88). The dashes are intentionally placed between the principles and modalities to indicate they are not separate. Many factors influence one's health. In recent years, particular attention has been paid to the influence

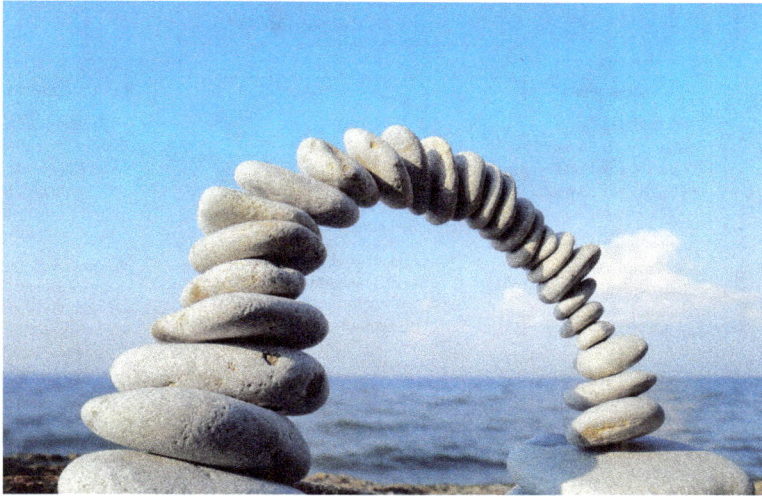

FIGURE 8.1   Arch of stones.

of social factors, including economics, culture, education, occupation and work setting, lifestyle, health care, relationships, and one's environment.

Well-being is used to describe a person's degree of holistic health. The AACN's definition was noted in the definitions section of this chapter. More recently, a concept analysis (Patrician et al., 2022) examined the well-being of nurses in depth. The results, including antecedents (or contributing factors), attributes (or characteristics), consequences (or outcomes) and definition, are depicted in the nurse well-being model (Figure 8.2).

Wellness is another abstract term closely related to well-being and is defined as "integrated, congruent functioning aimed toward reaching one's highest potential" (ANA 2015, p. 89). Does "highest potential" ring a bell? Right! It parallels self-actualization, the highest level of Maslow's hierarchy of needs (Mcleod, 2023). Sometimes wellness is used as a synonym for well-being. To be consistent, we will refer to *nurses' personal health and well-being.*

In surveys of nurses, the ANA (2016) has found that about two-thirds reported "putting the health, safety, and wellness of

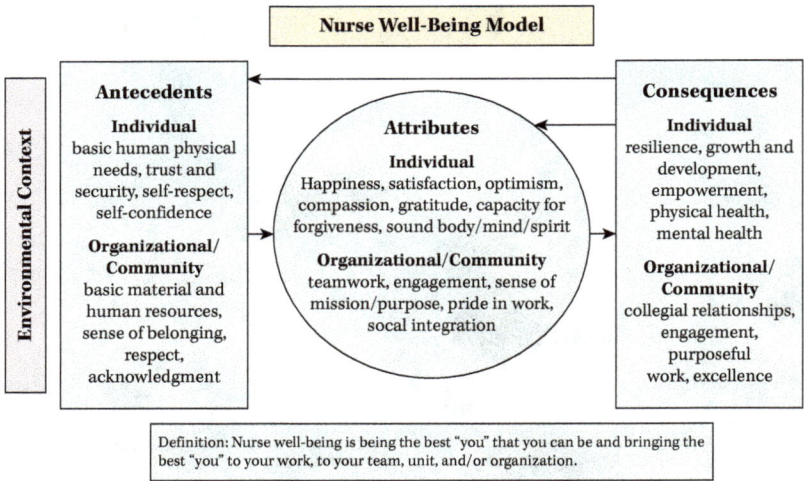

FIGURE 8.2 Nurse well-being model.

their patients before their own," (p. 4). When compared to the average American, nurses are more "likely to be overweight, have higher levels of stress and get less than the recommended hours of sleep" (ANA, 2023, para. 2). Nurses are also at high risk for injuries and illnesses that result in time off work (Dressner & Kissinger, 2018).

The COVID-19 pandemic increased nurses' stress and burnout, and their health and well-being declined. A 2021 study of over 264 nurses found over 50% reported worsening physical and emotional health relating to the pandemic. The ANF, in the *COVID-19 Two-Year Impact Assessment* (2022), reported that "60% of acute care nurses report feeling burned out, and 75% report feeling stressed, frustrated, and exhausted" (p. 1). Of particular concern were higher rates for nurses under 35. These findings don't just pertain to nurses in the United States. They are experienced by nurses and other health workers around the world (World Health Organization [WHO], 2022).

Although the body of research regarding the health and well-being of advanced nurses is less than that for RNs, there is evidence that advanced nurses are not immune to the stresses and strains of their work environment and are at risk for consequences such as burnout and moral distress (Prestia et al., 2017).

Physicians, pharmacists, and other health professionals are not immune to the negative outcomes, such as burnout, nurses have experienced due to the stresses and strains of the work environment (AMA, 2020; National Academy of Medicine [NAM], 2022). Later in this chapter, we'll discuss a national plan for improving the well-being of our health workforce.

Resilience

Resilience is a trait, process, or outcome (Reyes et al., 2015). It reflects the ability to adapt to challenges, stress, and adversity and to learn from it. Strategies to develop and internalize resilience can improve retention and reduce burnout. "Building positive relationships, maintaining positivity, developing emotional insight, creating work-life balance, and reflecting on successes and challenges are effective strategies for building resilience" (AACN, 2021, p. 63).

Stress that occurs in small amounts can be motivational and have a beneficial effect, but repeated or prolonged stress can negatively affect your health and well-being (Labrague & De Los Santos, 2020). Interventions designed to help individual nurses build their resilience and prevent or cope with burnout have been shown to support personal resilience in the short term (Henshall et al., 2020). However, as the Joint Commission (2019) notes, "Mindfulness and resilience training alone cannot effectively address burnout unless the leadership is simultaneously reducing and eliminating barriers and impediments to nursing workflow, such as staff and workplace environment concerns" (p. 2).

Much like the demands and stressors of the health care work environment, being a nursing student has stressors as well. Nursing students have a rigorous academic schedule. Worrying about grades and performance in the classroom, lab, and clinical setting contributes to student anxiety and stress. In addition to class, lab, and studying time, nursing students spend many hours each week in the clinical setting providing care in a complex and challenging environment and often have personal and work responsibilities outside of their education. Learning strategies to promote personal self-care can help students gain the knowledge, skills, and attitudes needed to better cope with the stress now and when they transition into practice in their new nursing roles.

Self-Care

Self-care is a process for which the aim or goal is improved health and well-being. The concept of self-care has a long history, having been noted by Socrates in Ancient Greece. However, formal use of the term *self-care* appeared in academic and then popular literature in the 1960s and '70s. Like health, well-being, and resilience, self-care is an abstract concept with many meanings. We offer two examples and a definition for this chapter.

One early use of the term came from nursing. In 1971, Dorthea Orem was a visionary nurse scholar who believed nursing should be an academic discipline and sought to identify how nursing was different from medicine and which aspects of health nurses could and should independently assess and manage. Orem suggested the concept of "self-care" belonged in nursing's "net" and defined self-care as "a human regulatory function that is a deliberate action to ensure the supply of necessary materials needed for continued life, growth, and development and maintenance of human integrity" (McEwen & Wills, 2019, p. 144).

Orem proposed three nested theories about self-care: self-care, self-care deficit, and nursing systems. Orem theorized that humans engage in self-care to the extent possible. A self-care deficit occurs when the person cannot fully care for themself. In that instance, nurses may intervene to provide the necessary care. Today, Orem's theories are integral to nursing practice in the United States and globally. They have been supported by a large body of research, adapted into middle-range and situation-specific theories, and used as the framework for curricula in nursing education programs and by health care organizations for nursing practice.

SELF-CARE BY NURSES

Self-care is a form of self-love that helps us maintain physical and mental fitness and promote personal resilience. The nurses' responsibility for self-care is a standard of professional nursing practice, addressed in the ANA Code of Ethics, and a strategy to help prevent and reduce the effects of today's health care environment. Self-care is not always an inherent skill; however, it can be cultivated over time.

Self-care is a process, whereas health, wellness, and well-being are outcomes perceived by the individual. Wellness and well-being are marked by emotional stability (e.g., coping effectively with life and creating satisfying relationships) and physical health (e.g., recognizing the need for physical activity, healthy foods, and sleep). A healthy lifestyle involves physical, mental, and social well-being (AACN, 2021, p. 59). Self-care and self-management are professional responsibilities to safe practice (ANA, 2001) and extend beyond safe practice to include nurses' satisfaction with a healthy work environment and personal health and well-being. Nurses should try to model the same health promotion they teach others. The standards of practice of the American Holistic Nursing Association (AHNA) include holistic nurse self-care; this core value refers to caring for self with regard to health and personal development. Caring for self involves the combination of holistic self-care practices and personal growth activities (Dossey et al., 2005).

Thoughts, feelings, and behaviors impact each other, influencing how we perceive life experiences (Figure 8.3). Our brains are

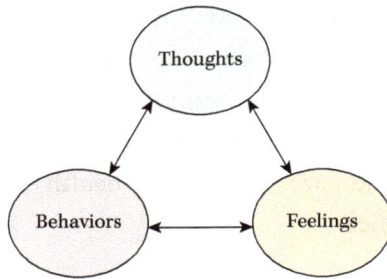

FIGURE 8.3   Relationship between thoughts, feelings, and behaviors.

wired to react more readily to negative thoughts that promote rumination, which engages us in repetitive negative thinking (Hanson, 2013). Stressors in the work environment are often taxing physically, emotionally, and spiritually and can affect nurses' well-being. The cumulative exposure to stress at work and the strain and stress of everyday life can affect nurses' professional and personal lives. Negative experiences and feelings in and about our work environment can lead to compassion fatigue, anxiety, burnout, turnover, and leaving the profession.

A proactive self-care routine has the power to boost your personal well-being and improve work performance, relationships, and physical health. Healthy nurses live life to the fullest capacity, as they become stronger role models, advocates, and educators in their community and work (ANA, 2023).

ADVANCED NURSES' SELF-CARE

A 2009 qualitative study of self-care among nurse leaders in a community hospital found that caring for oneself is part of life's journey (Brown, 2009). Many nurses, including advanced nurses, often experience challenges maintaining work-life balance and often put their patients, staff, and job responsibilities ahead of their own well-being. As leaders in their workplace, advanced nurses should be role models for colleagues and staff, including demonstrating self-care and supporting others so they can engage in self-care.

Maintaining work-life balance and personal self-care were challenges for advanced nurses pre-COVID-19, and they increased dramatically during the pandemic. In a 2021 survey, pediatric-focused APRNs in the United States reported that the COVID-19 pandemic had a negative impact on their personal and professional lives (clinical, education, and research). Among the APRNs surveyed, "34% reported moderate or extreme concern for feeling professionally burned out, 25% felt nervous or anxious, and 15% felt depressed or hopeless" (Peck & Sonney, 2021, p. 414).

While research on self-care by advanced nurses is limited, the topic has been addressed in columns by nurse leaders in journals and websites in the United States and other countries. The national president and national board director of the Australian College of Nurse Practitioners noted, "While we may take on some tasks traditionally only performed by medical officers, we maintain caring as our core role. But what happens when we run out of care? ... More than any single self-caring activity, a caring attitude or disposition towards oneself, rather than the archetypal self-sacrificing nurse, is the key to self-care" (Raftery & Poole, 2015, p. 653).

In the United States, nurses Leclerc et al. (2020) proposed a model of human-centered leadership that puts people first by making employee wellness a priority. They note findings from their research that "strong nursing leadership thrives on self-care nurse leaders advocating for their own self-care and encouraging their nurses to do the same" (p. 122). The roles of advanced nurses in promoting health and well-being in the workplace are discussed in more depth later in this chapter.

HOW TO PRACTICE SELF-CARE AND BUILD RESILIENCE

This section is designed to equip nurses with the skills to practice personal self-care, improve their resilience, and manage stress.

You will note that some activities overlap because they are part of self-care and help build resilience. Sometimes, people misunderstand what self-care involves. So, before you read on about strategies for personal self-care, look at Table 8.3 for some myths about self-care.

TABLE 8.3   **Top 3 Myths About Self-Care**

Self-care is selfish.	"Self-care is essential to affording us a life that reaches out to others and makes the world a better place. … You must care for yourself to care well for others" (Breakthrough, 2020, para. 8).
Self-care means becoming a yogi.	Self-care involves the person's holistic health. "It is not, by definition, limited to the physical self" (Breakthrough, 2020, para. 9).
I don't have time for self-care.	"Self-care isn't about adding to things to our lives. It can mean 'choosing to eliminate activities and responsibilities'; learning to say no. 'A little prevention in time and effort can make a significant difference in outcomes'" (Breakthrough, 2020, para. 10).

FIVE TYPES OF SELF-CARE

Self-care is a personal process in which individuals can choose activities based on their preferences, needs, and available resources. This chapter discusses five types of self-care: physical, emotional, social, mental, and spiritual attributes. Table 8.4 lists them and gives examples for each.

PHYSICAL

Physical self-care includes activities such as eating a healthy balanced diet, getting proper sleep, getting regular physical exercise, and managing your health. You will be less emotionally and mentally resilient if you do not meet your basic needs. Taking care of yourself increases your overall health and your sense of well-being. Choose physical activities you enjoy, such as walking, basketball,

TABLE 8.4 **Types of Self-Care**

Type	Examples of Activities
Physical	• Exercise for 30 minutes. • Walk with a friend. • Eat healthy foods.
Emotional	• Journal. • Practice gratitude; list two things each day that you are grateful for. • Schedule time for yourself on the calendar. • Declutter and get organized.
Social	• Limit social media time. • Spend quality time with a friend.
Mental	• Listen to music or podcasts. • Work on puzzles or play games.
Spiritual	• Meditate. • Pray. • Practice mindful breathing.

jogging, dancing, bicycling, yoga, tai chi, gardening, weightlifting, or swimming. The more you enjoy the activity, the more likely you are to continue doing it regularly. For example, working out with a friend often provides added motivation and commitment.

EMOTIONAL

Nurses typically put others' needs before their own. This can lead to neglecting emotional self-care. Practice self-compassion by placing your needs first. Schedule time for yourself on the calendar as you would any other appointment. Take time to observe your emotions in different situations to work on constructively expressing emotions. (Understanding your emotions is an important element of emotional intelligence; for more on emotional intelligence, see Chapter 2.) Use self-reflection, group work, or individual counseling to get comfortable with yourself and commit to self-care strategies. Journaling is an effective method that can help your emotional and mental well-being. Journaling can give you clarity of mind and increase focus to help you work effectively. Your thoughts and feelings are processed healthily through journaling, which can result in reduced stress (Walsh et al., 2020).

Rewiring our brains away from negative thoughts takes an intentional focus on gratitude and positive thinking. An intentional focus on positive thinking influences thoughts, feelings, and behaviors that help us change how we understand our experiences. Daily journaling and recording two positive thoughts helps to work on an intentional change from negative to positive thoughts, feelings, and behaviors and demonstrates healthy self-care behaviors that promote wellness and resiliency.

> Here are some examples of prompts you can use while journaling:
> 1. Write down thoughts, feelings, and behaviors that resulted from the day's experience.
> 2. Write down two positive things that went well today.
> 3. What challenges were presented?
> 4. What feelings can you recall having from the experience?
> 5. Reflect on how you responded to the events that happened during the day.

REFLECTION AND DEBRIEFING

Building the confidence and the skills needed to meet adversity takes time, experience, and practice. Reflection is a strategy that can help you grow your confidence, problem-solving skills, and resilience. Reflection allows individuals to identify and evaluate their own knowledge, skills, and beliefs. Reflection can be done individually or in a group discussion; however, it needs to be intentional and focused on encouraging thinking about concepts, gaining insight and knowledge, and developing self-awareness. Journaling is an example of individual reflection. Debriefing a simulation or an actual adverse event in the clinical or practice area is an example of a group reflection. Debriefing is a constructive reflective teaching strategy to give formative feedback, and it provides an opportunity to reflect on a situation to recount, describe, analyze, and reflect on situations. Debriefing is not an opportunity to point out poor behavior or decisions.

SOCIAL

Social media has provided a very easy connection to family, friends, and other followers. You have control over which accounts you follow, so follow accounts that provide positivity and unfriend those that make you unhappy. Limit the time connecting through social media and increase being with friends and family in person. Our busy lives make it challenging to make time to spend with family and friends, and it's often easy to neglect loved one's when our lives become busy. Close personal connections are important for our mental well-being. An intentional invitation to a friend or family member to spend time together is rewarding and meaningful.

MENTAL

How you think about different things affects your mind and dramatically influences your psychological well-being. Schedule time to do something that is of special interest to you. This keeps your mind engaged and enhances mental well-being. This might include listening to a podcast, painting, listening to music, building a puzzle, reading, or mindfulness meditation.

SPIRITUAL

The fifth type of self-care is spiritual, which connects us to something larger than ourselves. Spirituality, which is different from religion, can diversify thoughts to connect with one's true self and enhance inner calmness. This might include practices such as mindfulness meditation, prayer, religious rituals or services, spending time in nature, or engaging with art.

> Mindfulness is a practice that can help meet individuals' self-care needs through connection with themselves and others. Mindfulness encourages us to be more present and aware and helps us feel less overwhelmed. Mindfulness is something we are all capable of and it is easier to access when we practice it daily. It helps us to gain awareness of our emotional, mental, and physical processes (Mindful, 2023). Mindfulness meditation helps reduce feelings of anxiety and brings a sense of calm. Practicing 15 minutes of meditation will give you a sense of calmness, peace, and balance that can benefit your emotional well-being and your physical health. Slow, deep breathing can activate the parasympathetic nervous system, making you feel calm and safe (Hughes et al., 2021).
>
> Nurses can also practice brief periods of mindfulness during the workday. Stepping away from a stressful situation to sit in a quiet room and do a few minutes of slow, deep breathing can help the nurse be present and focus on the situation at hand. Being present can support effective clinical judgment as well as the nursing process, prevent adverse safety events, and build intentional, holistic caring relationships with patients.

WORK-LIFE BALANCE

"Work-life balance is the state of equilibrium where a person equally prioritizes the demands of one's career and the demands of one's personal life" (Sanfilippo, 2023). While it is important to acknowledge that there is no "perfect" work-life balance, here are some suggested strategies for promoting balance between your work and personal lives:

- Prioritize your health.
- Don't be afraid to unplug.

- Take a vacation.
- Make time for yourself and your loved ones.
- Set boundaries and work hours.
- Set goals and priorities and stick to them (Sanfilippo, 2023).

Reflection on Work-Life Balance

- What does work-life balance look like to you?
- Can you relate to the factors that impact work-life balance?
- Identify two strategies that you could work on to improve your work-life balance.

Advanced Nursing to Promote Self Care in the Workplace

Now is the time to educate nurses and employers on the importance of nurse self-care.

—ANA (2016, p. 6)

The AACN (2021) identified two advanced, system-level sub-competencies related to self-care: 10.1c, Contribute to an environment that promotes self-care, personal health, and well-being, and 10.1d, Evaluate the workplace environment to determine the level of health and well-being. In this section we will describe five approaches by which advanced nurses can promote and evaluate self-care in the health care work environment: (a) practice personal self-care, (b) role-model self-care, (c) lead system-based interventions in the workplace, (d) teach self-care within academic nursing education programs, and (e) lead or participate in initiatives by professional nursing organizations. By promoting self-care in the work environment, the advanced nurse will help promote the health and well-being of the nurses and other health care professionals who give so much of themselves every day.

Practice Personal Self-Care

It is essential that as leaders we model the self-care that replenishes and assures that we have the stamina in the long run. The first step is to make the commitment to self.

(Thompson, 2004, p. 197)

Recent literature, pre- and post pandemic, has addressed the importance of advanced nurses' self-care. For example, a study of nurses employed at the NIH (National Institutes of Health) Clinical Center in Maryland found that nurses, such as advanced nurses, who work outside of direct care are more likely to be sedentary and experience obesity (Ross et al., 2019). While all self-care activities in the section on nurses' personal self-care are relevant for advanced nurses, strategies have been identified specifically for advanced nurses. The following box indicates strategies suggested for Pediatric Nurse Practitioners but they have relevance for all advanced nurses (Gigli et al., 2022, p. 207).

Examples of Self-Care Strategies for APRNs

- Prioritize personal well-being.
- Seek mental health support and resources (e.g., mindfulness-based stress-reduction techniques, CBT, intentional gratitude).
- Commit to healthy lifestyle behaviors (e.g., limit alcohol intake, stop smoking, exercise regularly, eat a healthy diet, and prioritize sleep).
- Mindfully limit consumption of and exposure to news media and social media discussion forums.
- Seek mental health support early when symptoms first appear.

Role-Model Self-Care

By prioritizing their own health and well-being, nurse leaders are giving their staff permission to engage in their own self-care

—Ross et al. (2019, p. 606)

In their report of the NIH Clinical Center study, Ross et al. (2019) proposed that "one of the most important first steps managers can take to improve the health of their workforce is to reflect on their own patterns of activity, diet, and professional quality of life ... to better serve as role models for healthy living" (p. 9). An advanced nurse can model healthy behaviors in the workplace through activities such as eating nutritious meals away from the desk, taking breaks, avoiding extended time at work, and limiting emails at night or while on vacation (Ross et al., 2019).

When nurse leaders model self-care in the workplace, they are promoting self-care among their staff and implementing a core principle of leadership (Gächter & Renner, 2018). Perfection is not expected, but the advanced nurse should model consistent efforts to practice self-care and aim for work-life balance. Also, keep in mind that self-care is a journey; it is okay to acknowledge the ups and downs.

Systems-Based Practice to Promote Personal Self-Care in the Workplace

Systems-based practice, a competency of advanced nurses described in the AACN (2021) essentials domain 7, is "an analytical tool and a way of viewing the world, which can make caregiving and change efforts more successful. The focus is on understanding the interdependencies of a system or series of systems and the changes identified to improve the care that can be made and measured in the system" (p. 66). Figure 8.4 is one example of system-level models to illustrate the complexity of health and wellness at the system level (NASEM, 2019; NASEM, 2021).

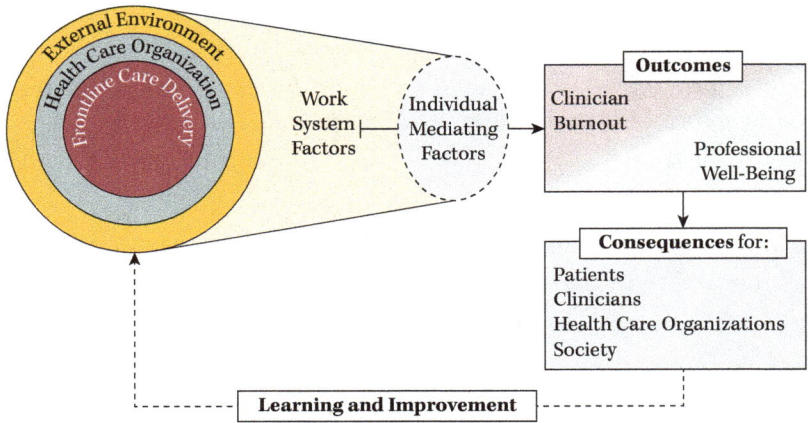

FIGURE 8.4 Systems model of burnout and well-being.

Advanced nurses can implement systems-based practice to lead projects or programs in their workplace designed to promote and support staff personal self-care and improve health, well-being, and resilience. In addition to the advanced competencies noted at the beginning of this section, the advanced nurse will also implement competencies from other AACN domains such as I, knowledge for nursing practice; III, population health; and VII, systems-based practice.

GETTING STARTED

Steps for leading programs to promote health and self-care for health care professionals:

1. In any improvement-type project, the first step is to form a planning committee of champions, stakeholders, and potential participants.

2. Next the committee "evaluates the workplace environment to determine the level of health and well-being" (AACN, 2021, p. 53). Elements assessed are tailored to the particular workplace setting but may include staff's perceptions of their personal health and well-being and that of the workplace

environment, the current level of self-care among the staff, outcomes of stressors of practice such as burnout and turnover, topics or services of interest to the staff, degree of senior leadership support, and available resources and assets within the organization for self-care programs. Keep in mind, the importance of staff health and well-being doesn't apply just to nurses. Programs described here can include everyone working in the identified workplace setting.

3. Strategies to gather the desired information should also be tailored to the workplace setting but may include forming subcommittees to promote engagement of additional staff and informal discussions with staff, surveys, or focus groups.

4. Led by the advanced nurse, the planning group uses models and theories of change and process improvement to frame one or more projects to promote staff self-care. Examples of such frameworks include the eight-step change process (Kotter, 2012) and the model for improvement (Institute for Healthcare Improvement, 2023). They may use different terms, but the components include planning, implementation, and evaluation. Depending on the advanced nurse's position and sphere of influence, these projects can be at three levels: microsystem, mesosystem, and macrosystem:

   - Microsystem: "Small, functional frontline units that provide the most health care to most people" (AACN, 2021, p. 61).
   - Mesosystem: "The interrelated parts and clinical leadership that provide care to certain populations" (AACN, 2021, p. 61).
   - Macrosystem: "The highest system level represents the whole of the organization and is led by senior leaders such as the CEO, chief operations officer (COO), chief nursing officer (CNO), chief information officer (CIO) and is guided by a board of trustees" (AACN, 2021, p. 61).

5. Plan and implement the program. In this phase, the advanced nurse leads the planning group to identify a goal,

outcome objectives, and specific elements of the project. A structure such as "who, what, where, when, and how" helps to prevent missing key details. A goal is a broad statement of the aim of the project, whereas outcome objectives are SMART: specific, measurable, achievable, relevant, and time bound (Minnesota Department of Health, 2023). The plan also includes a plan for evaluation. Examples of system-based projects to promote staff self-care are noted in Table 8.5.

6. Evaluate the program. It is important to evaluate any program or project designed to improve a situation in the health care setting. Evaluation should be planned prior to implementing the project and includes two foci and two timeframes: process (i.e., Did we implement our plan?) and outcome (Did we achieve our objectives? Did something change?). The timeframes are formative (during the project itself) and summative (after the project is completed). Process evaluation is formative and summative. Outcome evaluation is typically summative, and, for longer projects, it can also be formative with outcomes for phases of the project.

TABLE 8.5 **Levels of Health Care Systems and Examples of Self-Care Activities or Programs**

Level	Examples of Self-Care Activity or Program
All levels	• Model self-care. • Advocate for workplace programs to support staff self-care, resilience, and well-being. • Implement wellness advisory committees to provide input on staff burnout, turnover, and so forth and recommend and give feedback on programs to support staff health, resilience, and well-being. • Recognize and address factors influencing burnout, compassion fatigue, and turnover. Staff knowledge about self-care and resilience may not be enough (Ross et al., 2019).

Level	Examples of Self-Care Activity or Program
Microsystem	• Implement routine, brief (1–2 minute) breathing space or quiet time before report or meetings. • Designate space for meditation, reflection, or relaxation (i.e., sanctuary rooms, wobble rooms, serenity-lounge, Zen room, renewal room; Putrino et al., 2020) • Offer nutritious snacks at meetings instead of sugary treats. • Arrange for unit-based massage or yoga (Alexander, 2015). • Provide educational and support programs to build resilience (Blackburn et al., 2020; Kelly et al., 2021), prevent burnout (Couser et al., 2020), or address compassion fatigue (Adimando, 2017). • Provide mindfulness training.
Mesosystem	• Senior leaders advocate for, and support, activities at the microsystem level that meet staff-identified needs. • Be informed of complex factors influencing distress among staff, intent to stay (or leave), and turnover (see Figure 8.4). • Take action to acknowledge and address causes of distress (e.g., burnout) among nursing staff, promote job satisfaction, and reduce turnover (e.g., adequate staffing and staff empowerment). • Provide programs for nursing staff aimed at building mindfulness, ethical competence, and resilience through experiential and discovery learning, simulation, and communities of practice (National Academies of Sciences, Engineering, and Medicine, 2021).
Macrosystem	• Mission, vision, and strategic plan to prioritize and clearly communicate support for staff health and well-being. • Plan, implement, and evaluate corporate wellness programs (e.g., complementary health and well-being service; Hackman et al., 2023). • Communicate support for wellness programs (e.g., transparent participation by senior leaders, offering testimonials in meetings or through email, or leading a "wellness minute" in meetings; Aldana, 2023).

CONCLUSION

Nursing practice can have many rewards, both extrinsic (tangible rewards external to the job, e.g., salary and benefits) and intrinsic (intangible or psychological rewards, e.g., contributing to unit governance, progressing from novice to expert, and making a difference in people's lives). However, nurses also experience high levels of stress and strain due to complex, interacting factors such as the pace of health care, patient acuity, work schedules, and inadequate mix of numbers and skill levels of staff.

While nurses should look to their employers and professional organizations to address factors contributing to the high levels of stress and strain, they can implement self-care activities to promote their personal health, well-being, and resilience. The importance of these activities for nurses is acknowledged in numerous professional guides and programs such as the ANA code of ethics and Healthy Nurse, Healthy Nation (ANA Enterprise, 2021), the NAM (2022), and the WHO (2022). Moreover, they don't pertain just to nurses; self-care is a priority for all working in health care.

In this chapter, we identified the AACN competencies that pertain to nurses' self-care; provided background on health, well-being, resilience, and self-care; explained why they are important for nurses; and identified individual and system-level strategies that help nurses promote their personal health, well-being, and resilience. We also noted that, when implementing the advanced-level sub-competencies pertaining to self-care, nurses can also implement competencies from other domains.

KEY POINTS

- Self-care is a process or journey and, if managed well, can help promote your health and well-being.
- Self-care is not about being perfect. Do your best and be as compassionate with yourself as you are with your patients.

- Gratitude plays an important part in thoughts, feelings, and behaviors for positive thinking.
- A healthy lifestyle influences emotional stability and physical health for improved health and well-being.
- Health care organizations have a responsibility to implement strategies to provide healthy work environments and prevent burnout.
- Nurses who make their personal health and well-being a priority will be more resilient, able to cope with stressors at work, and attain work-life balance.
- Within health care organizations, advanced nurses can advocate for and lead
  - systems-based interventions to support nurses' self-care and, thus, their health, well-being, and resilience.
  - initiatives to address factors that contribute to the stresses and strains of nursing practice.

ACTIVITIES

Activity 1: Case Study—Stress Management

Jane is a senior in the final semester of an undergraduate nursing program. In the final 3 weeks of the semester, there are two major papers due and practicum hours to complete, in addition to being scheduled to work 20 hours per week at the local hospital where she is employed as a nursing assistant. After a disappointing grade on the midterm exam, Jane vowed to study weekly for the final but has not been able to do as much as she hoped. She paired up with a fellow classmate to help study for the final exam, but their schedules have not aligned to set up a time yet. Jane has been feeling a bit under the weather since returning from a 4-day trip home to attend a funeral service for a family member. There are only two planning meetings left to complete all of the activities for senior week. As chair of the planning committee, Jane has to finalize details for the food and decorations for the hall.

1. What is the issue?

2. What are the tasks that identify as stressors?

3. Brainstorm self-care strategies to minimize stressors in this situation.

4. List three activities that Jane can do to manage the upcoming final weeks of the semester.

Activity 2: Written Reflection on Self-Care

Think about a time you experienced a situation that led to stress and anxiety. This could be a conflict or situation resulting in stress in any setting (i.e., work, school, or a health care setting).

1. Describe the situation. What were the most important issues in the situation that lead to anxiety or stress?

2. What type of self-care practices did you use?

3. Do you think that stress levels were managed well? Why or why not?

Activity 3: Plan for Self-Care

Develop a personal plan for self-care.

1. Identify activities that support your health and well-being.

2. Set personal SMART goals: specific, measurable, attainable, relevant, and time-limited goals.

3. Write down one to two SMART goals for each of the five types of self-care.

Activity 4: Exploring Self-Care and Well-Being at the System Level

This activity can be done individually or in a small group.

1. Identify a business or organization. It could even be the college or university you attend.

2. Does the organization offer wellness or health-promotion activities? If so, what types? Check out the human resources website and talk with individuals who work there—family or friends or, if your school, faculty, and staff. Do they participate in the activities? How do they evaluate them? You could also talk with a staff person in the wellness program.

3. Write a summary of what you learned: what activities are offered, strengths, and so forth. How could they be improved?

Activity 5: Promoting Self-Care at the System Level

Complete this activity in a team of four learners.

1. Conduct an informal assessment of your peers regarding self-care. What does "mind-body" mean to them? What self-care activities do they do, how often, how do they feel after doing them, and do they help with their work or school experience? What challenges or barriers do they encounter in doing self-care? What resources do they use?

2. Plan and implement a self-care activity within your nursing program, such as yoga, mindfulness, gratitude, or walking. Have at least two measurable SMART goals: specific, measurable, attainable, relevant, and time limited.

3. Evaluate the activity with input from the planning group and participants: process (how it went and how many

people participated) and outcomes (if the objectives were met).

4. Write a brief report of the activity, including what went well and how could it be improved if done again.

REFERENCES

Adimando, A. (2017) Preventing and alleviating compassion fatigue through self-care: An educational workshop for nurses. *Journal of Holistic Nursing, 36*(4), 304–317. https://doi.org/10.1177/0898010117721581

Aldana, S. (2023). *7 ways how senior leaders can communicate support for the company wellness program.* https://www.wellsteps.com/blog/2022/07/21/communicate-support-company-wellness-program/

Alexander, G. (2015) Yoga for self-care and burnout prevention among nurses. *Workplace Health and Safety, 63*(10). https://doi.org/10.1177/2165079915596102

American Association of Critical Care Nurses. (2020) Recognize and address moral distress. https://www.aacn.org/clinical-resources/moral-distress

American Association of Colleges of Nursing. (2021). *The essentials: Core competencies for professional nursing education.* https://www.aacnnursing.org/AACNEssentials/Download

American Holistic Nurses Association. (2015). *Self-care and resilience.* https://www.ahna.org/American-Holistic-Nurses-Association/Resources/Self-Care-andResilience

American Medical Association. (2020) *Creating a resilient organization for health care workers during a crisis.* https://www.ama-assn.org/practice-management/sustainability/creating-resilient-organization-health-care-workers-during

American Nurses Association. (2001). *ANA code of ethics.* https://www.plu.edu/nursing/wp-content/uploads/sites/96/2014/10/ANA-Code-ofEthics.pdf

American Nurses Association. (2016). *Executive summary: American Nurses Association health risk appraisal.* https://www.nursingworld.org/~4aeeeb/globalassets/practiceandpolicy/work-environment/health–safety/ana-healthriskappraisalsummary_2013-2016.pdf

American Nurses Association. (2015). *Nursing: Scope and standards of practice* (3rd ed.).

American Nurses Foundation. (2022). *Pulse on the nation's nurses survey series: COVID-19 two-year impact assessment survey.* https://www.nursingworld.

org/~4a2260/contentassets/872ebb13c63f44f6b11a1bd0c74907c9/covid-19-two-year-impact-assessment-written-report-final.pdf

American Nurses Foundation. (2023). *Pulse on the nation's nurses: Three year annual assessment survey.* https://www.nursingworld.org/practice-policy/work-environment/health-safety/disaster-preparedness/coronavirus/what-you-need-to-know/annual-survey–third-year/

American Nurses Association. (2023). *Healthy nurse, healthy nation.* https://www.healthynursehealthynation.org/

Blackburn, L., Thompson, K., Frankenfield, R., Harding, A., & Linsdey, A. (2020). The THRIVE© program: Building oncology nurse resilience through self-care strategies. *Oncology Nursing Forum (ONF), 47(*1), E25–E34. https://doi.org/10.1188/20.ONF.E25-E34

Brown, C. (2009) Self-renewal in nursing leadership: The lived experience of caring for self. *Journal of Holistic Nursing, 27*(2), 75–84 https://doi.org/10.1177/0898010108330802

Breakthrough. (2020). *Self-care strategies: The top 3 myths about self-care.* https://www.break-through.ca/blogposts/science-of-self-care

Centers for Disease Control and Prevention. (2018). *Well-being concepts.* https://www.cdc.gov/hrqol/wellbeing.htm

Couser, G., Chesak, S., & Cutshall, S. (2020). Developing a course to promote self-care for nurses to address burnout. *The Online Journal of Issues in Nursing.* https://doi.org/10.3912/OJIN.Vol25No03PPT55

Dossey, B. M., Keegan, L., & Guzzetta, C. E. (2005). *Pocket guide for holistic nursing.* Jones & Bartlett Learning.

Dressner, M. A., & Kissinger, S. P. (2018). Occupational injuries and illnesses among registered nurses. *Monthly Labor Review*, 1–12.

Gachter, S., & Renner, E. (2018). Leaders as role models and "belief managers" in social dilemma. *Journal of Economic Behavior & Organization, 154*, 321–334. https://doi.org/10.1016/j.psychres.2020.112934

Gigli, K., Sonny, J., Lee, A., McNamara, M., Hunter, J., & Peck, J. (2022) Position statement on resilience and the postpandemic pediatric nurse practitioner workforce. *Journal of Pediatric Health Care, 36* (2), 205–209.

Hackman, E., Ryan, A., Lyons, L., Hopper, D., & Stringer, J. (2022). A model for staff support using complementary health and wellbeing. *Nursing Times, 118*, 11.

Hanson, R. (2013). *Hardwiring happiness* [Video]. TEDxvTalks. https://www.youtube.com/watch?v=jpuDyGgIeh0

Henshall, C., Davey, Z., & Jackson, D. (2020). Nursing resilience interventions—A way forward in challenging healthcare territories. *Journal of Clinical Nursing, 29*, 3597–3599.

Hughes, V., Cologer, S., Swoboda, S., & Rushton, C. (2021). Strengthening internal resources to promote resilience among prelicensure nursing students. *Journal of Professional Nursing, 37*(4), 777–783.

Institute for Healthcare Improvement. (2023). *Science of improvement: How to improve.* https://www.ihi.org/resources/Pages/HowtoImprove/ScienceofImprovementHowtoImprove.aspx

Joint Commission. (2019). Developing resilience to combat nurse burnout. *Quick Safety, 50.*

Kelly, F., Uys, M., Bezuidenhout, D., Mullane, S.L., & Briston, C. (2021). Improving healthcare worker resilience and well-being during COVID-19 using a self-directed e-learning intervention. *Frontiers in Psychology, 12,* 748133. https://doi.org/10.3389/fpsyg.2021.748133

Kotter, J. (2012). *Leading change.* Harvard Business Review Press.

Labrague, L. J., & De Los Santos, J. A. A. (2020). COVID-19 anxiety among front-line nurses: Predictive role of organisational support, personal resilience and social support. *Journal of Nursing Management, 28*(7), 1653–1661. https://doi.org/10.1111/jonm.13121

Leclerc, L., Kennedy, K., & Campis, S. (2020). Human-centered leadership in health care: An idea that's time has come. *Nursing Adminstration Quarterly, 44*(2), 117–126.

McEwen, M., & Wills, E. (2019). *Theoretical basis for nursing* (5th ed.). Wolters Kluwer.

Mcleod, S. (2023). *Maslow's hierarchy of needs.* Simply Psychology. https://www.simplypsychology.org/maslow.html

Medscape. (2022). *Medscape nurse career satisfaction report 2022: Contentment mixed with abuse and frustration.* https://www.medscape.com/slideshow/2022-nurse-careersatisfaction-6015927

Mindful. (2023). *What is mindfulness?* https://www.mindful.org/what-is-mindfulness/

Minnesota Department of Health. (2023). *Objectives and goals: Writing meaningful goals and SMART objectives.* https://www.health.state.mn.us/communities/practice/resources/phqitoolbox/objectives.html

National Academies of Sciences, Engineering, and Medicine [NASEM]. 2019. Taking action against clinician burnout: A systems apporach to professional well-being. Washington D.C.: The National Academies Press. doi: https://doi.org/10.17226/25521

National Academies of Sciences, Engineering, and Medicine. [NASEM] (2021). *The future of nursing 2020–2030: Charting a path to achieve health equity.* National Academies Press. https://doi.org/10.17226/25982

National Academy of Medicine. (2022). *National plan for health workforce well-being.* National Academies Press. https://doi.org/10.17226/26744

Newman-Bremang, K. (2021). *Reclaiming Audre Lorde's radical self-care.* Refinery 29. https://www.refinery29.com/en-us/2021/05/10493153/reclaiming-self-care-audre-lorde-black-women-community-care

Ohio League for Nursing. (2023). *2023 education summit handouts.* https://www.ohioleaguefornursing.org/page/2023SummitHa

Ohio Nurses Association. (2020). *The nurse wellness retreat.* https://ohnurses. org/wellnessconference/

Patrician, P., Bakerjian, D., Billings, R., Chenot, T., Hooper, V., Johnson, C.S., & Sables-Baus, S. (2022). Nurse well-being: A concept analysis. *Nursing Outlook, 70,* 639–650. DOI: 10.1016/j.outlook.2022.03.014

Peck, J., & Sonney, J. (2021) Exhausted and burned out: COVID-19 emerging impacts threaten the health of pediatric advanced practice registered nursing workforce. *Journal of Pediatric Health Care, 35*(4), 414–424.

Pender, N. (2011). *The health promotion manual.* https://deepblue.lib.umich. edu/handle/2027.42/85350

Porteous-Sebouhian, B. (2021, October 27). Why acknowledging and celebrating the Black feminist origins of "self-care" is essential. *Mental Health Today.* https://www.mentalhealthtoday.co.uk/blog/ awareness/why-acknowledging-and-celebrating-the-black-feminist-origins-of-self-care-is-essential

Prestia, A., Sherman, R., Demezier, C. (2017). Chief nursing officers' experiences with moral distress. *Journal of Nursing Administration, 47*(2), 101–107. https://doi.org/10.1097/NNA.0000000000000447

Putrino, D., Ripp, J., Herrera, J.E., Cortes, M., Kellner, C., Rizk, D., & Dams-O'Connor, K. (2020). Multisensory, nature-inspired recharge rooms yield short-term reductions in perceived stress among frontline healthcare workers. *Frontiers in Psychology, 11,* 560833 https://doi.org/10.3389/ fpsyg.2020.560833

Raftery, C., & Poole, L. (2015). Nurse practitioners: Do we care? *The Journal for Nurse Practitioners, 11*(6), 653. http://dx.doi.org/10.1016/ j.nurpra.2015.04.013

Reyes, A. T., Andrusyszyn, M. A., Iwasiw, C., Forchuk, C., & Babenko-Mould, Y. (2015). Nursing students' understanding and enactment of resilience: A grounded theory study. *Journal of Advanced Nursing, 71*(11), 2622–2633. https://doi.org/10.1111/jan.12730.

Ross, A., Yang, L., Wehrlen, L., Perez, A., Farmer, N., & Bevans, M. (2019). Nurses and health-promoting self-care: Do we practice what we preach? *Journal of Nursing Management, 27*(3), 599–608. https://doi.org/10.1111/ jonm.12718

Sanfilippo, M. (2023, October 23). How to improve your work-life balance today. *Business News Daily.* https://www.businessnewsdaily.com/5244-improve-work-life-balance-today.html

Thompson, P. (2004) Leadership from an international perspective. *Nursing Administration Quarterly, 28* (3), 191–198.

Walsh, P., Owen, P. A., Mustafa, N., & Beech, R. (2020). Learning and teaching approaches promoting resilience in student nurses: an integrated review of the literature. *Nurse Education in Practice, 45,* 102748.

World Health Organization. (2022). World failing in our "duty of care" to protect mental health and wellbeing of health and care workers finds report on impact of COVID-19. https://www.who.int/news/ item/05-10-2022-world-failing-in–our-duty-of-care–to-protect-mental-health-and-wellbeing-of-health-and-care-workers–finds-report-on-impact-of-covid-19#:~:text=The%20report%20found%20that%20 23,52%20percent%20in%20pooled%20estimates.

CREDITS

CHAPTER 9

Direct Observation of Team Interactions

Carol Savrin, DNP, CPNP, R, FNP-BC, FAANP, FANP, and Catherine Demko, PhD

KEY AACN COMPETENCIES, SUB-COMPETENCIES, AND CONCEPTS

Domain 6: Interprofessional Partnerships

Competency 6.2 Perform effectively in different team roles, using principles and values of team dynamics.

- ***Entry Level Sub-Competency 6.2a*** Apply principles of team dynamics, including team roles, to facilitate effective team functioning.

- ***Entry Level Sub-Competency 6.2b*** Delegate work to team members based on their roles and competency.

- ***Entry Level Sub-Competency 6.2c*** Engage in the work of the team as appropriate to one's scope of practice and competency.

- ***Entry Level Sub-Competency 6.2e*** Apply principles of team leadership and management. performance to improve quality and assure safety.

- ***Entry Level Sub-Competency 6.2f*** Evaluate performance of individual and team to improve quality and promote safety.

- ***Advanced Level Sub-Competency 6.2g*** Integrate evidence-based strategies and processes to improve team effectiveness and outcomes.

- ***Advanced Level Sub-Competency 6.2h*** Evaluate the impact of team dynamics and performance on desired outcomes.

Continued

Continued

- **Advanced Level Sub-Competency 6.2j** Foster positive team dynamics to strengthen desired outcomes.

KEY TERMS

Reflective listening	Psychological safety
Communication	Feedback: give and receive
Information	Situation monitoring
Collaborative	Team orientation
Team	Accountability
Mutual support	Adaptability
Leadership in teams	Team process

INTRODUCTION

Throughout this book there has been discussion of the American Association of Colleges of Nursing (AACN) 2021 competencies related to nursing in the interprofessional arena. AACN defines competency-based education as a system of instruction, assessment, feedback, and reflection. They also indicate that students need to understand their motivation, self-perceptions, and attitudes (AACN, 2023). In an effort to help students understand components of performance-based competencies for interprofessional teamwork and the corresponding evaluation of team function, the DOTI instrument was developed. As part of a Josiah Macy Jr. Foundation interprofessional grant, faculty from four disciplines (medicine, nursing, dental medicine, and social work) at Case Western Reserve University developed an instrument to assess the team interactions and team skills performance in the clinical setting. This instrument is called the DOTI (Direct Observation of Team Interactions) and was developed because it was determined that instruments available at the time were typically designed to measure specific behaviors in very specific clinical settings or had been intended for and utilized with experienced professional teams. DOTI was created to focus on the tasks and communications of health care teamwork with less emphasis on the specific clinical content or context of the interaction, potentially allowing its use in multiple settings (Brashers et al., 2019; Zorek et al., 2022). Further, the granular nature of the skill definitions is intended for early healthcare learners or anyone new to team dynamics. This chapter will discuss several ways this instrument can be used to assess team functioning as well as to teach the concepts of the competencies that are being assessed.

The DOTI instrument was created to define and standardize the assessment of team skills performance through the use of direct observation. Direct observation strengthens the assessment of interprofessional team learning beyond self-reported change and beyond basic knowledge and attitudes. The instrument includes 15 team skills organized in four domains (task communication, roles and leadership, interpersonal communication, and team process), with a five-point rating scale and anchor definitions for each behavior. In characterizing the team behaviors and defining the rating scale criteria, DOTI enhanced the detail and measurement of specific team skill behaviors to support learning as well as assessment.

DOTI's development drew on observable behaviors from the Interprofessional Education Collaborative's (IPEC) 2016 competencies and the Agency for Healthcare Research, Quality's (AHRQ, n.d.) TeamSTEPPS® teamwork system, simulation assessment methods (Rosen et al, 2010), and resources from the NEXUS interprofessional instrument collection (Brandt, 2017). The IPEC competencies were developed to help prepare future health professionals for team-based patient care and improved health outcomes. The goal of the IPEC competencies was to build on each profession's expected disciplinary competencies. The new AACN competencies include domain 6, interprofessional partnerships, to identify the collaborative skills nurses need to work with other health care professions to improve patient care. The AHRQ TeamSTEPPS® teamwork system was developed to enhance the function of teams in all settings. Utilization of the TeamSTEPPS® system promotes higher quality, safer patient care through a comprehensive curriculum fostering collaborative team skills in professional health care teams. Collaborative care skills in the final DOTI are similar to those of TeamSTEPPS® and the IPEC competencies and sub-competencies, including communication, leadership, situation monitoring, and mutual support. DOTI built on and operationalized the skill definitions for health professional students to enhance both learning and assessment. Among these and many other resources on interprofessional education and assessment, the general areas are very similar. All teams need practice and measurement in these areas to function as a team and improve the health care outcomes.

The DOTI instrument has been used for assessment of student team interactions in tabletop discussion cases, interprofessional team simulations with and without standardized patients, and authentic clinical settings, both inpatient and outpatient. In all of these settings, DOTI has demonstrated good to very good inter- and intra-rater reliability for observation in the hands of trained faculty, facilitators, and team coaches. The observed student teams generally consist of three to five early trainees from a variety of health professions, including nursing, medicine, dentistry, physician assistant programs, social work, and nutrition. DOTI served as both a framework for education and training in the collaborative team skills as well as for both formative and summative assessment. This intentional alignment of educational content and assessment measures through the use of DOTI can facilitate the student's appreciation and practice of the team skills. For example, formative assessment of and by the interprofessional team often led students to recognize the need for more critical self-assessment of both individual behaviors and team skills. For the purposes of this book, the competencies listed will be discussed and, in some cases, suggestions made for activities for each.

"Health care has not always been recognized as a team sport, as we have recently come to think of it. In the 'good old days,' people were cared for by one all-knowing doctor who lived in the community, visited the home, and was available to attend to needs at any time of day or night" (Institute of Medicine [IOM], 2012). Part of our responsibility now is to educate all health care students to understand the value and impact of team-based care. Health care providers must rely on others with greater expertise in order to provide the best evidence-based care for the patient. However, when relying on the expertise of others, there must be care coordination so that each of the providers is not working in a silo and is unaware of the activities of the others. Each health care profession has a different culture and environment. It is important that providers learn about the other professions' roles and cultures. When providing team-based care, there needs to be good communication, knowledge of the roles of others on the team helps to facilitate that. Understanding different language and culture can assist the team to be able to focus on the team itself. All of these activities can be monitored using the DOTI.

Much of what is called collaboration is more likely cooperation or coordination of care. Katzenbach and Smith (1993) argue that truly collaborative teams differ from high-functioning groups that have a defined leader and a set direction, but in which the dynamics of true teamwork are absent. The cases presented in this chapter exemplify why health professionals need to work in collaborative teams to ensure that care is accessible and patient centered (IOM, 2012).

In order to be successful, teams need a shared goal. Health care teams have a shared goal in the improved outcomes in patients. The team has a shared goal as well as shared responsibilities and interdependence. One aspect of the health care team that is a little different from other teams is the teams are often fluid or flexible. The physician working on the team today may not be the same next week. Similarly, the nurse may change day to day, but the goal of improved patient outcomes and professional membership remain stable.

COMPETENCIES

6.2a Apply principles of team dynamics, including team roles, to facilitate effective team functioning.

6.2c Engage in the work of the team as appropriate to one's scope of practice and competency.

Roles and responsibilities within a team will vary with the purpose, goal, and composition of the team. In health care, professional members will bring both unique and possibly overlapping scopes of practice with regard to patient care. (For more discussion of interprofessional roles, see Chapter 1 and Chapter 4.) Thus, strong organization, efficient communication, appropriate designation of roles, and shared, cooperative leadership will be necessary for effective team functioning. The roles members assume within the team refer not only to their clinical, patient-oriented tasks but very often to their roles and contributions to team meetings and huddles in order to develop and implement patient care plans. Often in health care, these roles change with each meeting and task that needs to be addressed. Shared vision, goals, and team priorities require a synthesis of input from all members, which contributes to their professional expertise. Nurses often have a variety of roles; they can be the case manager, they can be the caretaker, or they can be the primary care provider. Patients and other extended family also have a role, and the care team must work to engage them to effectively incorporate their attitudes, experiences, and preferences in health care decisions. Patient involvement will vary widely. Some patients will prefer to be very engaged in their care, while others will prefer to allow the health care team to manage their care. Likewise, some families are very involved in the care of their loved one, and others will step aside and allow the patient and the team to manage care. Monigle, in their *Humanizing Brand Experience*, identifies seven different types of patients from the "doctor dodgers" to the "habitual strugglers," to the "whole-health managers." The team has to be prepared to deal with all these different kind of patients when functioning in a team.

6.2b Delegate work to team members based on their roles and competency.

6.2e Apply principles of team leadership and management performance to improve quality and assure safety.

Leadership for effective interprofessional and interdisciplinary health care requires attention to the flattened hierarchy (i.e., a team in which each member contributes and is valued equally; Lake et al., 2020). In teamwork, leadership has often been described as "shared," meaning leaders guide, seek, and utilize group membership input to move the team process forward; they do not perceive or present themselves as sole authority. Leadership on IP teams may or may not be determined by authority or position; regardless, the leader must facilitate information sharing, collaborative decision-making, and psychological safety to create a climate of open communication that ensures quality and safe patient care. Team members have a responsibility here as well; they must professionally interact with leadership, cooperating when needed and challenging in instances of potential mistakes in patient care or team functioning. Shared leadership within a flattened hierarchy tolerates, actually encourages, these behaviors.

When one looks for information about roles within a team, one finds many different sources with many different roles (Lake et al., 2015, Lumen Learning, 2023; Marquis & Huston, 2020; Nelson et al., 2014; Weiss et al., 2018). In general, there is consensus that teams function more efficiently if there is a designated leader, someone focused on the tasks to be accomplished and someone focused on procedures. The health care team also has roles of various health care professions (nurse, pharmacist, physician, social worker, physical therapist etc.). On occasion, depending on the setting, a designated recorder is helpful when a team meeting occurs. There needs to be someone who keeps track of time (there is no setting in health care these days in which time is not of the essence). Often in health care, these roles change with each meeting and task that needs to be addressed. The most successful teams identify the roles at the beginning of the meeting.

DOTI FRAMEWORK AND DEFINITIONS

For roles and responsibilities, DOTI defines a high-functioning team as one that utilizes the professional and personal expertise of all members. There must be clarity in the assignment of responsibilities and honesty by members as to their professional skill and limitations so as to avoid unnecessary redundancy as well as gaps in care plans and care. If the team needs additional expertise, a plan exists to acquire such. Even on stable teams (i.e., those with recurrent members), roles may routinely change based on circumstance or purpose. For team discussion and rating, assessment should focus on identifying the skills and assets each member brings and if they are being appropriately utilized by the team.

For leadership, the DOTI criteria for a high-functioning team requires the behavior of shared, cooperative, collaborative, and empowering leadership. Strong leadership need not be diminished by sharing; in fact, the climate of shared leadership empowers others to demonstrate leadership skills, initiate topics for discussion, suggest solutions, and mediate team interactions if needed to ensure the goals of the team are met. Leadership on more stable teams may be systematically rotated or determined by "as-needed" situations. Expected leadership behaviors can and should be made explicit so that all members know them. For team discussion and ratings, assessment should focus on leadership's performance of (a) team tasks and procedures (staying on task, general team climate of professional interactions, team business such as scheduling, recording, attendance issues) and (b) cultivating "leadership behaviors" among the team members, empowering others to contribute and communicate as equals. Do members routinely and confidently introduce new ideas, identify barriers or gaps in team function, share information freely, ask questions without fear of reprisal? Clearly, leadership is primarily about ensuring that other teamwork behaviors are exhibited and fostered on the team.

Frank S., age 54, patient of the clinic. Frank lives alone (divorced), has two grown sons who live out of state. Frank's father has diabetes and has to have dialysis each week.

Jean M., NP, primary care provider

John K., social worker

Martin F., dentist

Janell C., nurse

Kristin S., pharmacist

Asafa A., physician

Vivy F., nurse navigator

SCENARIO 1

Frank comes to be seen in the clinic. He has not been seen for 3 years, as he lost his job during COVID and does not have health insurance. He presents today with increased fatigue, thirst, and urination. He has been getting up three or four times at night to urinate. In addition, he notes that his teeth are bleeding when he brushes his teeth. He has not seen a dentist in more than 5 years as he has not had any dental insurance.

Janell: "Jean, this next patient has a BMI of 30 and his BP today is 160/96. I think he is going to be a problem."

Jean: "Is he new to our clinic?"

Janell: "Yes, I think so, we do not have any history on him."

Jean enters exam room.

Jean: "Welcome Mr. S., may I call you Frank?"

Frank: "Yes."

Jean: "So you are here because of tiredness, thirst, and using the bathroom more often?"

Frank: "Yes."

Jean: "Do you have any thoughts on what might be causing this?"

Frank: "Well, I have been very stressed lately because I lost my job with COVID, and I have not been able to find a new one. I have no idea how I will pay for this visit."

Jean: "We might have ways to help you with that. Let's talk about the health concerns. Have you ever had any of these issues before?

Frank: "No, well, maybe the tiredness, but I really think that is from stress."

Jean: "I see that your father has diabetes, and I notice that your weight is rather high and your blood pressure was high today as well. Have you ever considered that you might have diabetes as well?"

Frank: "Oh, I am sure it is not that; I rarely eat any dessert or any sweet snacks. I usually have potato chips or crackers or pretzels."

Jean: "Well, diabetes can be a result of foods other than sweets; things like potato chips and other foods that have high carbohydrates, like pasta and bread, can be a problem as well. It is also much more common in people whose family members have diabetes as well. I think that we will do a glucose test today and see what that shows us if that is okay. In the meantime, I would like to have Janell take your blood pressure again and see what that is. I understand that you do not take any medications."

Frank: "No."

The NP leaves the exam room, and the nurse comes in.

Janell: "I am going to prick your finger and then recheck the blood pressure."

Jean does so and then leaves the exam room.

Janell (to Jean):   "The glucose is 256, and the BP now is 156/98."

Jean reenters the exam room.

Jean: "Frank, that glucose indicates that you have diabetes. Any number over 126, even if you just ate a meal, is too high. Your number was 256. We need to have you take some medications to bring that number down and also give you some meds to bring the blood pressure down. The high blood pressure can do damage to your heart and your kidneys. Bleeding gums can also be a sign of diabetes. We need to have you see a dentist to get the bleeding under control."

Frank: "There is no way that I can do all that. I have no insurance and cannot pay for medicines, much less a dentist. This will all just have to wait until I get a job. Oy, this is just one more thing to give me stress. I am sure that this is all just due to stress. Once I get a job, all this will go away."

Jean: "I am not sure that this will all go away once you get a job, and I do not want all of this to harm your body in the meantime. Let me have you talk to our social worker to see if you can get some assistance with your medical bills."

Frank: "Oh, all right, but I doubt that will help."

1. Are there any red flags here?
2. Does Frank understand the risk to his health?
3. Which health care personnel should be involved in Frank's care?
4. Would one expect all those providers to be in one location?
5. How does the nurse facilitate the collaboration of this team?
6. Who will most likely take the lead on this team?
7. Was Jean looking to promote positive outcomes for the patient?

Generally, most outpatient clinics do not have all of the services in one place. In some clinics there is a nurse who may be called a navigator to coordinate all the services. Whoever coordinates needs to have good communication skills and know and understand the different provider roles in order to facilitate the coordination of care. Most often a patient newly diagnosed with diabetes is going to need the services of a provider, potentially a pharmacist; all patients newly diagnosed with diabetes should see an ophthalmologist, and in this case Frank for sure needs to see a dentist as clearly his diabetes has affected his gum tissues. Because of his lack of insurance, Frank will likely need a social worker to facilitate the means for him to access care.

When a team works together to improve patient care, a variety of leadership styles might be employed to enhance the teamwork as well as the care of the patient. A servant or transformational leader will likely enhance patient care and improve team function.

TABLE 9.1 **Roles and Leadership**

Roles and responsibilities	Team roles and responsibilities are ignored and not well defined or underutilized. Members do not contribute their own knowledge or skills and ignore expertise and skills of other members.	1 2 3 4 5 N/A	Team recognizes, appreciates, and utilizes the roles of all its members. Members understand roles and responsibilities of others; recognize abilities and contribution from all members; and recognize their own limitations.
Mutual support	Team tolerates poor performance due to lack of support or do not assist each other when it is needed to accomplish the work.	1 2 3 4 5 N/A	Team encourages its members to support each other or ask for help. Team strives for high performance through assisting each other and compensates when members are overwhelmed; supports team focus.
Leadership	Team does not share leadership. Members are uncooperative with others' leadership. Team is often dominated by one member who limits discussion by imposing opinion.	1 2 3 4 5 N/A	Team demonstrates leadership appropriate for situation; members cooperate with shared leadership. Leader facilitates consensus and problem solving; provides statements of direction and empowers others; and facilitates team focus.

A laissez-faire leader or authoritarian leader will probably reduce productivity and may be a source of conflict. Contrary to what one might think, a visionary leader might not enhance team productivity. If the leader has ideas that are consistent with the rest of the team, the team can function very well, but if the leader has ideas that are not consistent, the team may not function well (Ronquillo et al., 2022).

With your classmates discuss these questions:

1. How will the nurse navigator organize this team?

2. Using the DOTI anchor definitions from the domain of roles and leadership, what should occur to indicate a high-functioning team?

3. What might occur to indicate a poor functioning team?

4. Who might best be the leader on this team?

5. What sort of leader might be best for this team?

SCENARIO 2

Entry Level Sub-Competency 6.2a: Apply Principles of Team Dynamics, Including Team Roles, to Facilitate Effective Team Functioning
Entry Level Sub-Competency 6.2e: Apply Principles of Team Leadership and Management Performance to Improve Quality and Assure Safety
Advanced Level Sub-Competency 6.2j: Foster Positive Team Dynamics to Strengthen Desired Outcomes

The clinic was able to get many members of the team together for a meeting. Team conference in conference room regarding Frank S.

Vivy F.: "I wanted to get everyone together so that I could have as much information as possible to try to work with Frank S. I understand that he was recently diagnosed with type II diabetes and that he currently is unemployed and has no insurance and has not followed through with the care that was prescribed. Is that about right?"

Janell: "Yeah, he was a real piece of work, refused to believe that he had diabetes despite being fat and then did not even call John to see if he could help with anything."

Jean: "Now, Janell, Frank was more upset about not having a job than about his diabetes, and we did not seem to be able to get him to understand that diabetes was a major problem."

Asafa A. "Why did you not have me see him? I would have made him understand."

Janell: "No one was going to get through to him!"

Jean: "Unfortunately we did not realize that we had not made him understand; maybe we should make another appointment and have him come in again."

Vivy F.: "Maybe it would be best if I went out and saw him at home. If he thinks that he will have to pay for another visit, he likely will not come."

Jean: "That is probably true, Vivy; that might be the best idea."

Martin: "You need to tell him that if he doesn't come and see me he will lose all his teeth."

Jean: "I do not think that is the best way to approach him."

Janell: "Well, he is not going to hear anything else!"

John: "I am going to need a lot of information to get him some help; maybe he would call me, if he will not come in."

Kristin: "He never filled his prescription, maybe if we went to metformin rather than the Ozempic, he could afford that."

Asafa A.: "I can't believe you put him on that drug, Jean. Why go with the designer drugs?"

Jean: "Those are recommended as firstline meds by the ADA, and his glucose was over 250."

Vivy: "So can we develop a plan if I am going to go out and try to work with him?"

1. Look at the roles and leadership categories of the DOTI. Which behaviors does each team member demonstrate from these 2 categories?
2. Did anyone take leadership role? If so, who?

3. Which behaviors in mutual support are demonstrated by team members?
4. Based on what you read, is this a high-functioning team?
5. If not, support your decision by identifying who and which behaviors were not contributing to team function.
6. Were any of the team members evaluating the impact of individuals on the team performance? If so, who?
7. How was the team promoting safety and quality?

When working in a team, all members of the team should be engaged in the process and should communicate clearly in order to facilitate the best outcome. In health care, the goal is to facilitate the best outcome for the patient. Look at the section of the DOTI related to interpersonal communication and the scenario. See if you can answer these questions.

6.2f Evaluate performance of individual and team to improve quality and promote safety.
6.2h Evaluate the impact of team dynamics and performance on desired outcomes.
6.2j Foster positive team dynamics to strengthen desired outcomes.

1. What type of feedback was given and was it appropriate in this situation?

2. How did the leader facilitate management to facilitate quality outcomes?

3. How did this team act to promote psychological safety?

4. How could the team have better responded to Janell and Asafa?

5. Do you think that the outcome for the patient is going to improve? Why or why not?

Some clinic settings are fortunate enough to have multiple health care personnel all in one clinic. If this is the case, a team can be brought together and can meet and discuss a complex case.

TABLE 9.2   **Interpersonal Communication**

Psychological safety	Team tolerates a lack of trustful relationships among members; members don't share their feelings, thoughts, or weaknesses with honesty.	1 2 3 4 5 N/A	Team supports its members to disclose feelings, weaknesses, and relevant experiences appropriately; trustful relationships are apparent through honest conversation, feedback, and questions.
Feedback: Give	The team tolerates feedback that criticizes, embarrasses, or blames. Giving feedback is avoided; members do not suggest improvement ideas.	1 2 3 4 5 N/A	Team feedback is constructive, empathetic, respectful, specific, honest, and nonjudgmental. Member feedback seeks to improve the team function and work goals. May be to team or individual.
Feedback: Receive	The team permits members to view appropriate feedback as criticism and become defensive, angry, or avoidant. Feedback ends on a negative note and learning opportunity is lost.	1 2 3 4 5 N/A	Feedback is appreciated and is used as an opportunity to learn or improve; members use feedback to be more effective.
Conflict management	The team avoids conflicts; disagreements are left unresolved before moving to another subject. Challenges are disrespectful.	1 2 3 4 5 N/A	Team demonstrates process to resolve differences of opinions and tasks; does not tolerate disrespectful or disruptive behavior that threatens team function; resolves differences positively.

Below is a complex patient and a discussion of a team meeting that occurred related to the patient. While the DOTI was developed specifically for use within teams, see if you think that any of the interpersonal communication skills might be useful in this patient scenario.

Together, these three competencies speak to the interactions among team members that impact the proximal outcome of high team functioning and the distal outcome of safe care and improved health outcomes. DOTI is focused on promoting and assessing the process of team functioning, without measures of patient health or safety. DOTI addresses these issues in three domains: task communication, interpersonal communication, and team process. The individual behaviors listed within each domain contribute to positive team dynamics. Assessment of these behaviors may be done as an individual or as a team, although DOTI was constructed to focus on team behavior. Individual self-assessment or even per assessment typically motivates students to practice and improve their own personal behaviors, thereby contributing more to the team function. Further, these assessments may be formative to help foster team dynamics by identifying what is being well done and what requires improvement. For stable teams with minimal personnel change, summative assessment using the rating scale can document a team's progress when compared to earlier assessments. Even dynamic health care teams generally have a stable purpose to achieve.

Two of the four DOTI domains define communication behaviors, as there is little doubt that poor communication among health care providers can compromise patient safety, care, and health outcomes (IOM, 2012). *Task communication* is concerned with exchanging information among team members, specifically the manner of delivering and receiving the information, the format, and the use of the information among the members. How a team member provides and receives information is a personal behavior, but how the *team* expects and tolerates the quality of those exchanges is how DOTI defines task communication. Further, DOTI prompts evaluation on the engagement of team members ensuring that all contribute and all are heard. Finally, how the team uses that information in the collaborative decisions impacts patient care.

One of the main functions of task communication is *clearly* sharing information with other members of the team. Often, different health care professionals use different terminology for the same idea (in nursing, students practice skills in a clinical rotation, whereas in social work, they practice their skills in a structured practicum). This is just one example of different terminology. Part of task communication is the respectful sharing of terminology and active listening on the part of the members of the team. When working in an interprofessional team, the members have to trust that the other health care providers are going to carry out their designated function (task). Respect is a large part of task communication and underlies all interactions with the team.

TABLE 9.3   **Task Communication**

	Low		**High**
Reflective listening	Team tolerates members interrupting, side conversations, or members ignoring each other.	1 2 3 4 5 N/A	The team expects members to listen without interruption and be attentive to whomever is speaking. Members demonstrate listening by asking questions or participating; nonverbal cues, eye contact, body language.
Team dialogue/ engagement	The team ignores poor participation by members; tolerates withdrawal from discussions.	1 2 3 4 5 N/A	The team expects and supports all of its members to engage in meaningful discussion. All members participate in discussions and are engaged in dialogue.

	Low		**High**
Information sharing	Team permits members to not share information that is clear, relevant, or timely. Members do not explain professional terminology.	1 2 3 4 5 N/A	Team insists on members sharing appropriate information that is clear, sufficient, organized, and relevant. Members check for understanding; practice SBAR process.
Collaborative decision-making	Team tolerates unilateral decision-making. The problem-solving and decision processes are not inclusive; different opinions are not sought or are ignored.	1 2 3 4 5 N/A	Team seeks input and incorporates all the different perspectives in the decision-making process. Final decisions are a synthesis of ideas, perspectives, and expertise.

Interpersonal communication defines how information is shared and how professional relationships are managed and maintained in the team. Along with team process, these are the two DOTI domains that capture the core of team dynamics and require the most attention to achieve a high-functioning team. The ability to speak and question freely without the fear of rebuke or reprimand is essential. Nonjudgmental, constructive feedback, given and received in the spirit of team improvement, is the basis for addressing and resolving conflict. These behaviors have trust at their core, which means they typically take time to develop and require consistent nurturing. These sections can have guidelines that must be adhered to and communicated to new team members as needed, and if the guidelines are not strong it leaves the team vulnerable to mistakes and gaps in patient care and safety.

Poor communication among clinicians and resulting disparities in care priorities have been well documented. Effective communication between clinicians is vital to improve patient care. A CRICO study (2016) indicated that of 23,000 malpractice suits, more than 7,000 could be directly attributed to lack of communication.

TABLE 9.4 **Interpersonal Communication**

Psychological safety	Team tolerates a lack of trustful relationships among members; members don't share their feelings, thoughts, or weaknesses with honesty.	1 2 3 4 5 N/A	Team supports its members to disclose feelings, weakness, and relevant experiences appropriately; trustful relationships are apparent through honest conversation, and feedback, questions.
Feedback: Give	The team tolerates feedback that criticizes, embarrasses, or blames. Giving feedback is avoided; members do not suggest improvement ideas.	1 2 3 4 5 N/A	Team feedback is constructive, empathetic, respectful, specific, honest, and nonjudgmental. Member feedback seeks to improve the team function and work goals. May be to team or individual.
Feedback: Receive	The team permits members to view appropriate feedback as criticism and become defensive, angry, or avoidant. Feedback ends on a negative note and learning opportunity is lost.	1 2 3 4 5 N/A	Feedback is appreciated and is used as an opportunity to learn or improve; members use feedback to be more effective.
Conflict management	The team avoids conflicts; disagreements are left unresolved before moving to another subject. Challenges are disrespectful.	1 2 3 4 5 N/A	Team demonstrates process to resolve differences of opinions and tasks. Does not tolerate disrespectful or disruptive behavior that threatens team function; resolves differences positively.

SCENARIO 3

Mr. M, 64 years old, is brought to the ED by his ex-wife. Mr. M. called his ex-wife, and according to her was talking gibberish and she was concerned that he was having a stroke. She drove to his home, picked him up, and took him to the ED. Mr. M was admitted to the hospital for evaluation of a potential stroke and further medical evaluation. Upon exam it was determined that his electrolytes were very abnormal. His sodium and chlorine were very elevated, and his calcium and potassium were low. His electrolytes were stabilized in the hospital, and his medications were renewed and several were changed. He was discharged home after 4 days.

Mr. M and his ex-wife are in the exam room. Mina Green, NP, enters exam room.

Mina: "Mr. M, I see that you are here for follow-up after your hospitalization. How have things been going since you got home?"

Mr. M: "Okay, I guess. I still can't get around very well but otherwise okay."

Mina: "You say you cannot get around; why is that?"

Mr. M: "Well, since my stroke I have to use this walker, and I can't drive, so I am pretty much stuck at home."

Mina: "How do you manage to get groceries and things?"

Mrs. M: "Oh, I stop by and bring him his groceries and take him to appointments and so forth."

Mina: "That is very kind of you. So, Mr. M, what medications are you taking now?"

Mr. M: "Oh, well, I take the water pill and the pink one for my blood pressure, and I use the inhaler."

Mina: "Did you get new ones from the hospital?"

Mr. M: "No, they gave me some prescriptions, but I have not been able to fill them, and I don't know what they are for anyway."

Janice, the front office person, knocks and comes in.

Janice: "I just got a fax from the hospital. There are a whole bunch of new meds on here. Mr. M, you really need to get them if you want to stay out of the hospital again.

Mina: "Thanks Janice."

Mr. M: "How am I supposed to do that? I can't get out."

Janice: "Well, you need to figure out a way."

Mina: "Thank you, Janice, that will be all."

He has several diagnoses, including chronic obstructive pulmonary disease, hypertension, prior stroke, decreased mobility likely due to prior stroke, and now the electrolyte imbalance. He lives alone. He has not been eating well, his ex-wife takes him to the grocery store on occasion, but he does not often get healthy food and then is not taking the time to prepare meals. Additionally, because of his previous stroke, his mobility is impaired, and he uses a walker. He admits that he spends most of the day sitting in a chair and watching TV.

1. Which aspects of Mr. M's care require a team approach?
2. Which team members should be involved in the care?
3. Do you think that Janice displayed any negative (or positive) interpersonal communication issues from the DOTI?
4. How could the situation have been addressed better than it was?
5. Who might best lead the team care for this gentleman?
6. If you were leading the team, what would be your first priority, and what team member would you contact to address this priority?

Because of the complexity of Mr. M's case, it was decided that a team of health care professionals was needed. The team needed the NP, the pharmacist, a nutritionist, a social worker, and a physical therapist. The team will need to work together to address all of Mr. M's varied issues.

SCENARIO 4

The team that was put together consisted of

Nurse	Jenna
Nurse practitioner (provider)	Mina
Clinical pharmacist	Cindy
Social worker	Scott
Physical therapist	Shoshana

The team met and the NP described the patient as indicated.

Scott: "What a mess!"

Mina: "Surely we can find some way to help this patient."

Cindy: "Well, there is not much I can do without a complete list of his medications. I also need to know what he is taking and what he is not."

Mina: "This is what they faxed over from the hospital, but it is not clear to me that everything is there, because his antihypertensive, which he is taking, is not listed. There does not seem to be anything for hypertension."

Jenna: "Well, I can call the hospital and see if I can get this cleared up. I have no idea why we always get these confusing records. Don't they realize that we need *everything*, not just the new ones?"

Mina: "Scott, do you think that you could call Meals on Wheels and get him some regular meals? He was hospitalized with electrolyte imbalance, and if he does not eat regular meals he will end up back there."

Scott: "Well, I can try, but they are really not doing much now. They apparently have a hard time getting folks to deliver, so they are only taking people who cannot get out at all, and from what you said, he does get out."

Mina: "He gets out, but on a very limited basis and not to get groceries or meals. Please try, this really is for the patient's best outcome."

Scott: "All right, but don't blame me if it does not happen."

Mina: "Shoshanna, do you think that you could make a home visit to get him started on some physical therapy?"

Shoshanna: "Considering our workload now, no one would be able to get out there for maybe 3 weeks. We might have someone who could go then."

Mina: "Is there no way you could get out there sooner?

Shoshanna: "No, there is no way! We could fit him in here if he came in here."

Mina: "Maybe I will ask if the ex-wife could bring him in here."

Cindy: "So if I get that list, what do you want me to do with it?"

Mina: "If we have to have him come in for the physical therapy, maybe you could talk to him about his meds at the same time."

Cindy: "I can try, but if he doesn't fill them and doesn't want to take them, what can I do?"

Jenna: "If we can get this all coordinated, I can join you and explain the importance of all those meds along with what you are telling him."

1. Was this meeting productive? Why or why not?
2. practicing good interpersonal communication?
3. Which, if any, of the participants demonstrated good task communication?
4. Who could improve in either category?
5. Did the leader have good control? Why or why not?
6. How would you suggest improving the meeting?

The final domain of the DOTI is team process, which aims to synthesize individual member behaviors into a cohesive team identity and behavior, which should exceed the sum of its parts (i.e., individual member behaviors). Team process is comprised of the action team members take to combine their individual resources, knowledge, and skill to resolve their task demands and achieve collective goals. The team process involves setting team goals, which in turn relates back to task communication. The team members have to be accountable for their respective responsibilities, and there needs to be adaptability, because often in health care, team members change and new members join. Team process includes all of these activities and is vital to the positive functioning of a team. Teams consist of a variety of personality types, and each personality tends to work differently in a team setting (Resick et al., 2014). An individual may initiate situation monitoring, calling attention to poor team performance in some, but the team must respond. Individual members may be accountable and adaptable regarding their assigned tasks, but does the team exhibit the qualities in their performance?

TABLE 9.5   **Team Process Section of DOTI**

Team situation monitoring	Team ignores poor team functioning. Members do not speak up about conflict, misunderstandings, tension, or inability to get work done.	1 2 3 4 5 N/A	Members speak up and acknowledge the need for action when team functioning is threatened or concern is expressed about team performance. Members monitor/recognize/correct team process and functioning as a whole.
Team orientation	Team allows the members to focus on individual goals above team goals. Members make remarks that individual expertise could reach effective conclusions alone.	1 2 3 4 5 N/A	Team establishes integrated team goals over only individual professional focus and goals. Includes patient voice as needed. Team demonstrates need for multiple perspectives and expertise in person-centered, safe care.
Accountability	Team tolerates a lack of accountability. Members have negative responses to being held accountable for tasks and behaviors.	1 2 3 4 5 N/A	Team follows up on assigned tasks. Reminds each other of agreed-on duties and cooperates to be accountable.
Adaptability	Team appears unwilling or unable to change processes or roles as needed; members articulate unwillingness to change. Change disrupts functioning.	1 2 3 4 5 N/A	Team changes or improves the way work is accomplished as needed. Team recognizes and openly discusses need and process for change; members appear to have confidence in the team to change and adapt.

Using the team meeting described earlier, rank each of the communication skills above based on what you read. Then discuss with your classmates what the positive and negative points indicated. In addition, discuss the roles as indicated in the prior DOTI list.

1. How were health care providers used appropriately?
2. Did the different health care providers display appropriate roles?
3. Was there respect for the various roles that were represented?
4. How was there collaborative decision-making exhibited?
5. Did someone appear to be the leader?
6. How did the leader facilitate consensus or not?

Nurses are integral members of interprofessional health teams in all settings for patient care. Their contributions to the team will vary among direct clinical care, administrative services, care coordination, and many others, often assuming a leadership role in the team. Nurses' communication skills combined with clinical expertise and teamwork experience can promote high-functionating health teams that ensure optimal patient care and safety. Team skills exemplified by the DOTI instrument provide a framework to foster the development and implementation of these skills in both educational and practice settings. Consistent, intentional practice of these skills in both simulated and clinical settings will help nurses develop the required competencies to fully participate in effective, efficient team-based care.

REFERENCES

Agency for Healthcare Research and Quality. (n.d.). *TeamSTEPPS*. https://www.ahrq.gov/teamstepps/index.html

American Association of Colleges of Nursing. (2021). *The essentials: Core competencies for professional nursing education.*

Brandt B.F., Schmitz C.C. (2017). The US National Center for Interprofessional Practice and Education Measurement and Assessment Collection, *Journal of Interprofessional Care, 31*(3), 277–281.

American Association of Colleges of Nursing. (2023). *What students need to know about the AACN essentials.*

Brashers, V., Haizlip, J., & Owen, J. A. (2019). The ASPIRE model: Grounding the IPEC core competencies for interprofessional practice within a foundational framework, *Journal of Interprofessional Care, 34*(1), 128–132.

CRICO (2016) Press rerelease: Failures in communication contribute to medical malpractice. https://www.rmf.harvard.edu/news-and-blog/press-releases-home/press-releases//2016/february/failures-in-communication-contribute-to-medical-malpractice/

Institute of Medicine. (2012). *The future of nursing: Advancing health.*

Interprofessional Education Collaborative. (2021). *Core competencies for interprofessional collaborative practice.*

Katzenbach, J., and Smith, D. (1993). The discipline of teams. *Harvard Business Review*, March-April.

Lake, D., Baerg, K., & Paslowski, T. (2015). *Teamwork, leadership and communication.* Brush Education.

Luebbers, E. (2021). *Web-based toolkit to guide implementation of IPE in the clinical setting.* National Center for Interprofessional Practice and Education. https://nexusipe.org/informing/resource-center/web-based-toolkit-guide-implementation-ipe-clinical-setting

Lumen Learning. (2023). *Creating effective teams.* https://courses.lumenlearning.com/wm-organizationalbehavior/chapter/creating-effective-teams/

Marquis, B., & Huston, C. (2021). *Leadership roles and management functions in nursing: Theory and application.* Wolters Kluwer.

Monigle. (2023). *Humanizing brand experience.* https://www2.monigle.com/hbe-vol6-report.

Nelson, S., Tassone, M., & Hodges, B. (2014). *Creating the health care team of the future: The Toronto model for interprofessional education and practice.* Cornell University Press.

Resick, C. J., Murase, T., Randall, K. R., & DeChurch, L. A. (2014). Information elaboration and team performance: Examining the psychological origins and environmental contingencies. *Organizational Behavior and Human Decision Processes, 24*(2), 165–176.

Ronquillo, Y., Ellis, V. L., & Toney-Butler, T. J. (2022). *Conflict management. StatPearls.* https://www.ncbi.nlm.nih.gov/books/NBK470432/

Rosen M.A., Weaver, S.J., Lazzara E., Salas E., Wu T., Silverstri, S., Schiebel N., Almeida S., and King, H.B. (2010). Tools for evaluating team performance in simulation-based training. *Journal of Emergency Trauma Shock, 3*(4), 353–359.

Weiss, D., Tilin, F., & Morgan, M. (2018). *The interprofessional health care team.* Jones and Bartlett Learning.

Zorek, J. A., Ragucci, K., Eickoff, J., Najjar, G., Ballard, J., Blue, A.V., Bronastein, L., Dow, A., Gunaldo, T. P., Hageman, H., Karpa, K., Michale, B., Nickol, D., Odiaga, J., Ohtake, P., Pfeifle, A., Southerland, J. H., Vlasses, F., Young, V., & Zomorodi, M. (2022). Development and validation of the IPEC Institutional Assessment Instrument. *Journal of Interprofessional Education and Practice, 29*(12). https://www.sciencedirect.com/science/article/pii/S240545262200060X

APPENDIX: DOTI FORMS

Direct Observation of Team Interactions (DOTI)
Full Reference Guide

Instructions: Use a 5-point scale to rate how the team generally performed the behavior during the observation period. Anchor definitions are provided. NA if behavior is not needed and not observed.

		LOW		HIGH
		TASK COMMUNICATION		
REFLECTIVE LISTENING	Team tolerates members interrupting, side conversations, or members ignoring each other.	1 2 3 4 5 NA		The team expects members to listen without interruption and be attentive to whomever is speaking. Members demonstrate listening by asking questions or participating; nonverbal cues, eye contact, body language.
TEAM DIALOGUE/ ENGAGEMENT	The team ignores poor participation by members; tolerates withdrawal from discussions.	1 2 3 4 5 NA		The team expects and supports all of its members to engage in meaningful discussion. All members participate in discussions and are engaged in dialogue.
INFORMATION SHARING	Team permits members to not share information that is clear, relevant or timely. Members do not explain professional terminology.	1 2 3 4 5 NA		Team insists on members sharing appropriate information that is clear, sufficient, organized and relevant. Members check for understanding; practice SBAR process.
COLLABORATIVE DECISION-MAKING	Team tolerates unilateral decision-making. The problem-solving and decision processes are not inclusive; different opinions are not sought or are ignored.	1 2 3 4 5 NA		Team seeks input and incorporates all the different perspectives in the decision-making process. Final decisions are a synthesis of ideas, perspectives and expertise.
		ROLES AND LEADERSHIP		

	LOW		**HIGH**
ROLES & RESPONSIBILITIES	Team roles and responsibilities are ignored, not well defined, or underutilized. Members do not contribute their own knowledge or skills and ignore expertise and skills of other members.	1 2 3 4 5 NA	Team recognizes, appreciates and utilizes the roles of all its members. Members understand roles and responsibilities of others; recognize abilities and contribution from all members; recognize own limitations.
MUTUAL SUPPORT	Team tolerates poor performance due to lack of support of each other. Members do not provide support or assist each other when it is needed to accomplish the work.	1 2 3 4 5 NA	Team encourages its members to support each other or ask for help. Team strives for high performance through assisting each other and compensates when members are overwhelmed; supports team focus.
LEADERSHIP	Team does not share leadership. Members are uncooperative with other's leadership. Team is often dominated by one member who limits discussion by imposing opinion.	1 2 3 4 5 NA	Team demonstrates leadership appropriate for situation; members cooperate with shared leadership. Leader facilitates consensus and problem solving; provides statements of direction and empowers others; facilitates team focus.
INTERPERSONAL COMMUNICATION			
PSYCHOLOGICAL SAFETY	Team tolerates a lack of trustful relationships among members; members don't share their feelings, thoughts, or weaknesses with honesty.	1 2 3 4 5 NA	Team supports its members to disclose feelings, weakness, and relevant experiences appropriately; trustful relationships are apparent through honest conversation, feedback, questions.
FEEDBACK: GIVE	The team tolerates feedback that criticizes, embarrasses or blames. Giving feedback is avoided; members do not suggest improvement ideas.	1 2 3 4 5 NA	Team feedback is constructive, empathetic, respectful, specific, honest and nonjudgmental. Member feedback seeks to improve the team function and work goals. May be to team or individual.

(Continued)

	LOW		HIGH
FEEDBACK: RECEIVE	The team permits members to view appropriate feedback as criticism and become defensive, angry, or avoidant. Feedback ends on a negative note and learning opportunity is lost.	1 2 3 4 5 NA	Feedback is appreciated and is used as an opportunity to learn or improve; members use feedback to be more effective.
CONFLICT MANAGEMENT	The team avoids conflicts; disagreements are left unresolved before moving to another subject. Challenges are disrespectful.	1 2 3 4 5 NA	Team demonstrates process to resolve differences of opinions and tasks. Does not tolerate disrespectful or disruptive behavior that threatens team function; resolves differences positively.
TEAM PROCESS			
TEAM SITUATION MONITORING	Team ignores poor team functioning. Members do not speak up about conflict, misunderstandings, tension, or inability to get work done.	1 2 3 4 5 NA	Members speak up and acknowledge the need for action when team functioning is threatened or concern is expressed about team performance. Members monitor/ recognize/ correct team process and functioning as a whole.
TEAM ORIENTATION	Team allows the members to focus on individual goals above team goals. Members make remarks that individual expertise could reach effective conclusions alone.	1 2 3 4 5 NA	Team establishes integrated team goals over only individual professional focus and goals. Includes patient voice as needed. Team demonstrates need for multiple perspectives and expertise in person-centered, safe care.
ACCOUNTABILITY	Team tolerates a lack of accountability. Members have negative responses to being held accountable for tasks and behaviors.	1 2 3 4 5 NA	Team follows up on assigned tasks. Reminds each other of agreed-upon duties and cooperates to be accountable.

	LOW		**HIGH**
ADAPTABILITY	Team appears unwilling or unable to change processes or roles as needed; members articulate unwillingness to change. Change disrupts functioning.	1 2 3 4 5 NA	Team changes or improves the way work is accomplished as needed. Team recognizes and openly discusses need and process for change; members appear to have confidence in the team to change and adapt.

Interprofessional Learning, Experience, and Practice (ILEAP), "Direct Observation of Team Interactions (DOTI)," 2016–2020 ILEAP Project Toolkit and Guide. Copyright © by Case Western Reserve University. Reprinted with permission

DOTI Abbreviated Reference Form With Rating Scale

	LOW	**HIGH**
TASK COMMUNICATION		
REFLECTIVE LISTENING	Interrupting, side conversations	Attentive; asking questions or participating; eye contact, acknowledgments
TEAM DIALOGUE/ ENGAGEMENT	Poor participation in discussions	Meaningful discussion. All members participate
INFORMATION SHARING	Information unclear, uses discipline-specific vocabulary without explaining	Share information; clear, sufficient, organized. SBAR when appropriate
COLLABORATIVE DECISION-MAKING	Decisions not inclusive	Final decisions synthesize ideas; all have opportunity for input
ROLES AND LEADERSHIP		
ROLES & RESPONSIBILI-TIES	R&R underutilized; professional perspectives ignored	Team utilizes professional roles and responsibilities of all
MUTUAL SUPPORT	Poor support or assist when needed	Assisting each other; compensates when members are overwhelmed/not present
LEADERSHIP	Leadership not shared; inappropriate dominance tolerated	Leadership shared; members cooperate with appropriate leadership; leader facilitates team focus
INTERPERSONAL COMMUNICATION		
PSYCHOLOGICAL SAFETY	Don't share feelings, thoughts, or weaknesses with honesty	Trustful relationships apparent; honest conversation, feedback, questions

(Continued)

FEEDBACK: GIVE	Team tolerates critical/ judgmental feedback; feedback does not offer improvement ideas	Feedback is constructive, specific, nonjudgmental; improves the team function; situation appropriate for team or individual
FEEDBACK: RECEIVE	Recipient gets defensive; ends on negative note	Feedback used as opportunity for team improvement; facilitates self-assessment
CONFLICT MANAGEMENT	Conflicts/ disagreements left unresolved	Team demonstrates process to resolve differences positively

TEAM PROCESS		
TEAM SITUATION MONITORING	Ignores poor team functioning. Members do not speak up	Need for action is addressed through team tools; members monitor/recognize/correct team functioning
TEAM ORIENTATION	Individual goals more than team goals	Members voice value of multiple perspectives and expertise
ACCOUNTABILITY	Team tolerates lack of accountability	Follows up on tasks. Reminds team and individuals
ADAPTABILITY	Fails to recognize required or potential for positive change; unwilling/unable to change	Recognize and discuss needed change; open discussion to change processes

RATING SCALE				
1. Routine uncorrected poor behaviors; no team correction; no skill criteria met; needs significant improvement	2. Few positive behaviors; few skill criteria met; mostly uncorrected poor skills; needs improvement; not acceptable	3. Mixed; some poor, some positive; attempts to correct not fully effective; acceptable as a novice team	4. Frequent positive behaviors; most skill criteria present; no overt poor skill; developing skill; solid, mostly strong	5. Consistent, advanced positive behaviors; exemplify high functioning team on this behavior; all skill criteria present; excellent, strong behavior

Interprofessional Learning, Experience, and Practice (ILEAP), "DOTI Abbreviated Reference Form with Rating Scale," 2016–2020 ILEAP Project Toolkit and Guide. Copyright © by Case Western Reserve University. Reprinted with permission.

DOTI Comment and Rating Form

Team ID:	Observer ID:	Date:	Time:	
	RATINGS **LO HI**			
TASK COMMUNICATION				
REFLECTIVE LISTENING	1 2 3 4 5 NA			
TEAM DIALOGUE/ ENGAGEMENT	1 2 3 4 5 NA			
INFORMATION SHARING	1 2 3 4 5 NA			
COLLABORATIVE DECISION-MAKING	1 2 3 4 5 NA			
ROLES AND LEADERSHIP				
ROLES & RESPONSIBILITIES	1 2 3 4 5 NA			
MUTUAL SUPPORT	1 2 3 4 5 NA			
LEADERSHIP	1 2 3 4 5 NA			
INTERPERSONAL COMMUNICATION				
PSYCHOLOGICAL SAFETY	1 2 3 4 5 NA			
FEEDBACK: GIVE	1 2 3 4 5 NA			
FEEDBACK: RECEIVE	1 2 3 4 5 NA			
CONFLICT MANAGEMENT	1 2 3 4 5 NA			

(Continued)

TEAM PROCESS		
SITUATION MONITORING	1 2 3 4 5 NA	
TEAM ORIENTATION	1 2 3 4 5 NA	
ACCOUNTABILITY	1 2 3 4 5 NA	
ADAPTABILITY	1 2 3 4 5 NA	
Interprofessional Learning, Experience, and Practice (ILEAP), "DOTI Comment and Rating Form," 2016–2020 ILEAP Project Toolkit and Guide. Copyright © by Case Western Reserve University. Reprinted with permission.		

INDEX